KU-012-744

THE
LITTLE
BOOK
OF
MEDICAL
BREAKTHROUGHS

DR NAOMI CRAFT

NEW
HOLLAND

For Saul, Natasha and Isaac.

Published in 2008 by New Holland Publishers (UK) Ltd
London • Cape Town • Sydney • Auckland
www.newhollandpublishers.com
Garfield House, 86–88 Edgware Road, London W2 2EA, United Kingdom
80 McKenzie Street, Cape Town 8001, South Africa
Unit 1, 66 Gibbes Street, Chatswood, NSW 2067, Australia
218 Lake Road, Northcote, Auckland, New Zealand

10 9 8 7 6 5 4 3 2 1

ISBN 978 1 84773 068 8

Publishing Director: Rosemary Wilkinson
Editors: Giselle Osbourne; Julia Shone; Aruna Vasudevan
Editorial Assistant: Nicole Whitton
Design: Focus Publishing, Sevenoaks, Kent and Phil Kay, New Holland
Illustrator: Heather McMillan
Production: Melanie Dowland
Reproduction by Pica Digital Pte. Ltd., Singapore
Printed and bound in India by Replika Press

The paper used to produce this book is sourced from sustainable forests.

Contents

HOW TO USE THIS BOOK

The New Holland Little Books are easy-to-use comprehensive guides to important subjects. The Little Books feature over 100 entries on key principles or theories essential to understanding the subject. Written in an easily accessible manner, each Little Book explains sometimes very difficult concepts and theories, putting them in their historical context, giving background information on the experts who proposed them in the first place, analysing influences and proposing, where relevant, links to other related entries. The books also feature tables, equations and illustrations, and end with a glossary, where relevant, and an index.

The Little Book of Medical Breakthroughs is arranged chronologically and the country of origin is listed, where appropriate. Each entry includes a clear main heading, the person or people responsible for the discovery, birth and death dates, where relevant, followed by a short introductory paragraph explaining the concept concisely. In some cases, the main essay is also cross referenced to linked subjects. The book ends with a comprehensive index.

Other books in the series include: *The Little Book of Environmental Principles* and *The Little Book of Mathematical Principles*.

The name of the medical breakthrough

The year or years of discovery, followed by the country or countries of discovery.

The name or names of the person or persons responsible for the breakthrough, followed by their birth and death dates (where relevant).

A brief summary of the breakthrough.

A concise one- to three-page entry, explaining the medical innovation's importance and putting it in context.

Some entries are supported by explanatory diagrams, illustrations or photographs.

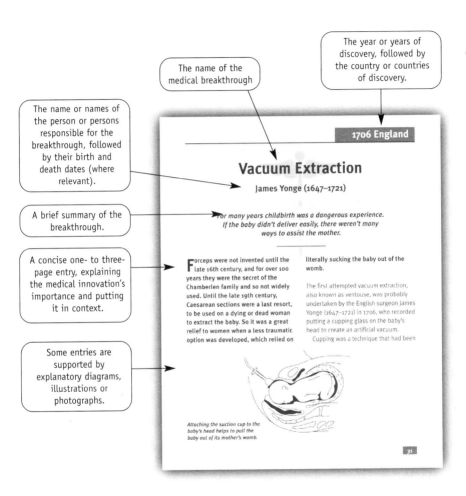

Vacuum Extraction

James Yonge (1647–1721)

For many years childbirth was a dangerous experience. If the baby didn't deliver easily, there weren't many ways to assist the mother.

Forceps were not invented until the late 16th century, and for over 100 years they were the secret of the Chamberlen family and so not widely used. Until the late 19th century, Caesarean sections were a last resort, to be used on a dying or dead woman to extract the baby. So it was a great relief to women when a less traumatic option was developed, which relied on literally sucking the baby out of the womb.

The first attempted vacuum extraction, also known as ventouse, was probably undertaken by the English surgeon James Yonge (1647–1721) in 1706, who recorded putting a cupping glass on the baby's head to create an artificial vacuum.

Cupping was a technique that had been

Attaching the suction cup to the baby's head helps to pull the baby out of its mother's womb.

31

Glass Eyes

Although known as glass eyes, artificial eyes are now made out of plastic, and are often so lifelike that they cannot be distinguished from the normal eye.

The oldest-known artificial eye was found in 2006 in the remains of a young woman living nearly 7,000 years ago – around the time of the Ancient Greeks – in what is now Iran in the Burnt City historical site.

It was probably made of natural tar mixed with animal fat. The thinnest blood vessels on the eyeball were made with golden wires, less than a millimetre thick. The eyeball had two holes on its two sides for fixing the eyeball to the socket.

Most Ancient Egyptian artificial eyes were made out of enamelled metal or painted clay attached to cloth and worn outside the socket. These were known as Ectblepharons. Not much changed over the next 10 centuries. Writing in the 16th century, French surgeon Ambrose Paré (1510–1590) described gold or silver versions, worn in front of the eyelids when they were known as *ekblephara* and under the eyelids when they were known as *hypoblephara*.

Late in the 16th century, false eyes began to be made out of enamel and glass. Exactly who made the first glass eye is not known, but the English playwright William Shakespeare (1564–1616) knew about them when he wrote in *King Lear*:

> *Get three glass eyes;*
> *And, like a scurvy politician, seem*
> *To see the things thou dost not.*
> –King Lear to the Earl of Gloucester, Act IV, Scene 6

The first English artificial eyemaker set up business in Ludgate Hill in London in 1681, advertising enamel artificial eyes, '*so exact as to seem natural*'. Enamel was attractive but expensive and didn't last long. More popular were glass eyes.

Initially the Venetians, famous for glass making, were the main glass eye makers. However, by the mid 19th century, the experts in glass eye making mostly came from a region of Eastern Germany called Thuringia. Their products were of such high quality that they became popular all over the world. German craftsmen known as ocularists toured the United States custom-making artificial eyes, stopping for a few days in each city, fitting patients for new eyes, before moving on to the next. Fabricating secrets were closely guarded, passed down from one generation to the next. Eyes were also fitted by mail order. An ocularist would also keep hundreds of pre-made eyes, which were cheaper, providing patients with the closest fit.

Since the Second World War (1939–1945), plastic has become the preferred material for making artificial eyes. There is no risk of breaking, chipping or scratching. A plastic eye can be more easily moulded to irregular contours of the eye socket, and can be worn all the time instead of having to be removed at night.

Sutures

A surgical suture is used to stitch together the edges of a wound after an operation or to repair damaged tissue.

Some sutures dissolve, others don't. They can be man made or natural (from silk, linen and catgut). Some are made out of one single filament, which causes less damage to the tissues but are harder to knot, or several filaments that are braided or twisted together.

Some of man's earliest records show evidence of sutures. We know needles were used at least 3,000 years ago and archaeological records from ancient Egypt show that the Egyptians used linen and animal sinew to close wounds. In ancient India, physicians used the heads of beetles or ants to staple wounds shut. The live creatures clamped the edges of the wound shut with their pincers. Then their bodies were twisted off, leaving their heads in place. Other natural materials used by doctors in ancient times included flax, hair, grass, cotton, silk, pig bristles and animal gut.

The first description of catgut was in 175 AD. Made from sheep intestine (and bearing no relation to cats) this was easily available from musicians who used it for strings.

Not much progress was made in the use of sutures until the 19th century, when surgery became a viable option with the invention of adequate anaesthesia. Although surgery was less painful, wound infections were a major cause of death. Sutured wounds seemed more likely to become infected, so many surgeons preferred not to use them.

In 1847, the Viennese obstetrician Ignaz Semmelweis (1818–1865) discovered that handwashing considerably reduced the risk of infection, making surgery much safer. Having realized the benefit of disinfectant, Joseph Lister (1827–1912) Professor of Surgery in Glasgow, Scotland, used carbolic acid to clean his hands and instruments, and also soaked his catgut sutures in it. The infection rate fell dramatically and carbolic-soaked catgut became widely accepted by 1860.

As well as his contribution to antisepsis, Lister was the first to discover that the body absorbed catgut sutures. Absorbable sutures are useful for a wound that doesn't need to be supported for more than a few days. Lister realized that if he soaked his sutures in chromic acid, like the tanners who used it to soak their leather, the catgut would last a week or longer. In 1881 chromic catgut was introduced.

By 1890 the catgut industry was firmly established in Germany, thanks to its use in the manufacture of sausages. From 1906 it was also sterilized using iodine.

Catgut was the staple absorbable suture material through the 1930s and, at one stage, one of the major manufacturers of catgut sutures, Ethicon, reported using intestines of 26,000 sheep a day! Where a non-absorbable material was needed, surgeons continued to use silk and cotton. Suture technology advanced with the creation of nylon and polyester in the late 1930s. Needle technology also advanced and surgeons began using a needle which was crimped onto the suture, therefore reducing the trauma to the wound because the needle and the suture were the same width.

In the 1960s chemists developed new synthetic materials that could be absorbed by the body, such as polyglycolic acid and polylactic acid, and better sterilization technology, so that sutures could be sealed in a package and then sterilized, as they are today.

See: *General Anaesthetic*, pages 48–49; *Handwashing*, page 72; *Sanitation*, pages 61–62

Artificial Limbs

For as long as people have been losing limbs there have been attempts to make artificial ones. A prosthesis is a replacement for a limb (or part of a limb) that has been amputated or may have been missing from birth.

The first known description of a prosthetic limb is in the *Rig-Veda*, an ancient Indian sacred poem written in Sanskrit between 3500 and 1800 BC. The story is about a warrior, Queen Vishpla, who lost her leg in battle. Once she had been fitted with an iron prosthesis, she was able to return to the fight.

Probably the oldest actual example of a prosthesis is the Cairo toe. It was found attached to the foot of an ancient Egyptian mummy dating from between 1069–664 BC. It is made of leather and wood, and is flexible. It looks worn, suggesting it was used, and not just added after death. Scientists believe the woman was in her mid-50s and may have lost the big toe from complications of diabetes.

Older still is the Greville Chester Great Toe, named after the man who acquired

it for the British Museum, which dates between 1295 and 664 BC. It is made of linen glue and plaster blended together, but this one doesn't bend and was probably cosmetic.

Before the Egyptian toes were discovered, the oldest prosthesis in existence was the Roman Capua Leg, which was found in a grave in Capua, Italy, dating to 300 BC. It was made of bronze, but unfortunately it was destroyed during an air raid in the Second World War. A copy is kept at the Science Museum in London.

Generally, early prostheses didn't have much function. Pliny the Elder (23–79 AD), a 1st-century Roman scholar, described a typical prosthesis when he wrote about Marcus Sergius, a Roman general who had his right arm amputated in the battle against Carthage (c. 218–210 BC).

To allow him to get back to battle, Pliny writes that the general had an iron hand made by his armourer just to hold his shield in place. Others describe artificial legs that fitted into the stirrups allowing a soldier to balance on a horse, but not enabling them to walk.

In the 16th century, French Surgeon Ambrose Paré (1510–1590) started developing prosthetic limbs with basic functionality. 'Le Petit Lorrain' was a hand operated by springs and catches for a French army captain. He also invented an above-knee prosthesis, which consisted of a peg leg with a foot prosthesis. It had an adjustable system for attaching it to the body, knee-lock control and other engineering features.

By the 19th century, there had been more advances and greater attempts to make limbs more functional. For example, Douglas Bly of Rochester, New York, invented and patented 'Doctor Bly's anatomical leg' in 1858. As Bly commented, this one still had its limitations:

'Though the perfection of my anatomical leg is truly wonderful, I do not want every awkward, big-fatted or gamble-shanked person

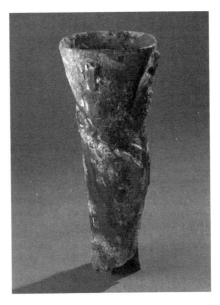

A copy of an artificial leg in brass and plaster made around 1910 from the original at the Royal College of Surgeons, London. The original was found in a Roman grave in Capua, Italy.

who always strided or shuffled along in a slouching manner with both his natural legs to think that one of these must necessarily transform him or his movements into specimens of symmetry, neatness and beauty as if by magic – as Cinderella's frogs were turned into sprightly coachmen.'

In recent years, there has been more emphasis on developing artificial limbs that look and move more like actual human limbs. Advances in biomechanics, engineering and plastics, combined with the use of computer-aided design and computer-aided manufacturing, have all contributed to the development of more realistic artificial limbs.

One of the latest inventions in this field includes the world's first commercially available bionic hand, which has five individually powered digits. To work it relies on the electrical signal generated by muscles in the remaining part of the patient's limb to open and close the fingers. Electrodes sitting on the surface of the skin pick up the signals.

One of the first patients to be fitted with the bionic hand summarized the significance of the development when he said:

'It's truly incredible to see the fingers moving and gripping around objects that I haven't been able to pick up before. The hand does feel like a real replacement for my missing hand.'

Urinalysis

Studying urine has been part of medical diagnosis for thousands of years. Initially all there was to go on was the colour, smell, and even taste. Fortunately, now we have more sophisticated methods to help identify infections, chemicals and crystals.

Ancient Chinese and Indian records mention observations of the urine from 1000–2000 BC. But the most detailed information we have comes from Hippocrates (c. 460–c. 375 BC), the apocryphal 'father of modern medicine' who wrote about urine examination in 400 BC. He observed the different smells and colours of urine. During Hippocrates's lifetime, it was common practice to pour a sample of urine on the ground to see if it attracted insects. If it did, it was called 'honey urine' – later known as diabetes.

Urine examination was developed further in 1000 AD, by a Peruvian physician called Abu Ibrahim Ismail al-Jurjani (1045–1137) who not only noted that it was possible to observe the smell and colour of the urine, as Hippocrates had observed, but also its quantity, consistency, transparency, sediment and froth.

In the Middle Ages, physicians became known as uroscopists because of their ability to examine urine. Typically the sick patient's servant would bring a urine sample to the physician, and leave it for analysis – for a fee.

Several physicians were consulted, and they would compete to get the most accurate (or possibly the most attractive diagnosis) by wheedling information out

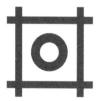

Before written language, symbols were used to represent natural elements, and this was the ancient symbol for urine.

of the servants – often by giving them a drink or two. The physician who did best would get to look after the patient – and therefore a greater fee.

Charlatans went one step further, claiming to be able to tell the future based on examination of the urine. They were known as 'Pisse Prophets', and brought the practice of uroscopy into disrepute.

In the 17th century the English physician Thomas Willis (1621–1675) advocated tasting urine to detect the sweetness caused by diabetes. It wasn't until 1776 that Matthew Dobson (1731–1784), a Liverpudlian physician, evaporated urine from diabetics and found that it left a residue that smelled and tasted like sugar.

Fortunately in the 18th century several tests were developed for testing specific chemicals in urine, including protein and sugar. However, it wasn't until 1956 that the first test strip for analyzing urine was introduced.

Condoms

In the 21st century we have easy access to cheap, single-use polyurethane condoms.

Condoms have been around since Ancient Greek times, although not in their present form. The Greeks used linen ones which, although unreliable, were perhaps more appealing than the tortoiseshell ones that the Japanese favoured, or the leather, animal gut or fish bladder condoms used at different times around the world.

In the 1500s when writing about the prevention of syphilis, the Italian anatomist Gabrielle Fallopio (c. 1522–1562) recommended wearing his invention – a linen sheath over the glans, but under the foreskin, or inserted into the urethra. A more practical version described later by Italian practitioner Hercules Saxonia (1551–1607) involved a larger linen sheath, soaked in a chemical or herbal preparation, which covered the entire penis.

The name condom probably comes from *Condus*, the Latin for receptacle.

There is also an alternative explanation, probably apocryphal, that in the 1600s the physician of English king Charles II (1630–1685) was called Dr Condom, or Quondam. Allegedly, the doctor made sheaths of oiled animal gut to protect the king from syphilis.

Condoms made from sheep's intestine were more widely available in the 1700s. The gut was soaked, turned inside out, macerated in an alkaline solution, scraped, exposed to brimstone vapour, washed, blown up, dried, cut and given a ribbon tie. This labour-intensive process meant that the result was quite expensive, so they were often reused and only available to a limited proportion of the population.

In 1843 rubber vulcanization, invented by Charles Goodyear (1800–1860) and Thomas Hancock (1823–1871), made it possible to produce cheaper, more reliable condoms that were stretchier and easier to use. However, men were still encouraged to wash and reuse them.

The manufacture and supply of condoms changed radically in the 1930s with the development of liquid latex condoms, superseding rubber completely. Prices plummeted and mass production began. By the mid 1930s, the 15 largest makers in the United States were producing 1.5 million condoms a day.

Since then, new technology has improved the condom considerably. The Durex Avanti, launched in 1994, is made from a unique polyurethane material, DURON, which is twice as strong as latex, enabling a thinner, more sensitive film.

Caesarean Section

The operation to remove a child from its mother's womb to save the baby's life was a breakthrough. However, when it was first introduced, it was only done when the mother was dead or dying. It was in effect a medical failure for the woman. The first successful Caesarean in Britain did not take place until the late 19th century.

Caesareans have been carried out since Ancient times. Apollo removed Asclepius from his mother's womb according to Greek myth, and there are many references to the operation in ancient Hindu, Egyptian, Greek, Roman and other European folklore.

The origin of the word 'Caesarean' is unclear. In 7th century BC the Romans passed a law – the *Lex Caesara* – stating that all pregnant women dying while in labour should have surgery to remove the baby. Popular myth suggests that Julius Caesar (100–44 BC) was born this way, although this seems unlikely, because history records that his mother Aurelia (120–54 BC) lived on to see her son's invasion of Britain. The word may also originate from the Latin verb *caedare* that means to cut, or possibly from the word *caesones*, the name given to infants who were cut from their mother's womb.

The word 'section' comes from the surgical term, which means to divide tissue. In a Caesarean, the wall of the abdomen and uterus are both divided to get the baby out.

A Caesarean was a last resort, and nobody really expected the baby to survive, let alone the mother. This began to change in the 19th century, when doctors began to learn more about the anatomy of the body and so were more likely to be successful if they operated.

New developments in antisepsis meant that women were less likely to die from infection after a surgical procedure. Anaesthetics were developed which transformed the experience for the woman. Whereas in the past surgeons had been afraid to sew up the cut in the uterus because they thought internal stitches might cause infection and a ruptured uterus in subsequent pregnancies, by the late 1880s sutures were commonplace.

As the operation became less risky, obstetricians began to recommend the procedure at an earlier stage, rather than waiting until the baby and mother were almost dead, when their chances of surviving any surgical procedure were limited.

The first recorded Caesarean in which both mother and child survived was probably carried out some time in the late 19th century.

See: *General Anaesthetic,* pages 48–49; *Sanitation*, pages 61–62

Spectacles

The invention of spectacles transformed life from a shapeless blur to sharp focus for many people. It is not clear exactly when they were invented or by whom, but certainly they were in use by the end of the 13th century.

Although there were no spectacles in Ancient times, there were certainly many people with poor vision. Famously, Marcus Tullius Cicero (106–43 BC), the Roman philosopher and orator, wrote to his friend Titus Pomponius Atticus (c. 110–32 BC), one of Rome's great writers and statesmen, saying that his slaves had to read to him because he could no longer read to himself now that he was old.

Allegedly there was an alternative even in Roman times: the Roman philosopher and dramatist Lucius Annaeus Seneca (4 BC–65 AD) claims to have read '*all the books in Rome*' by looking through a glass bowl filled with water, which would have acted as a primitive lens.

The theoretical principles behind corrective lenses were already in place, as we have evidence that the Greek astronomer Ptolemy (85–165 AD) had

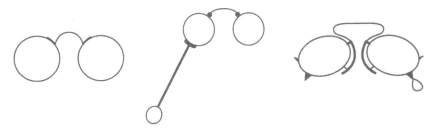

The above illustrations shows a selection of early spectacles.

described the basic laws of diffraction in roughly 140 AD. However, it wasn't until the 17th century that these laws were formalized and developed further by Willebrord Snellius (1580–1626), a Dutch astronomer and mathematician.

Reading stones, often made from quartz, became popular in the 8th century, first in Spain and spreading to the rest of Europe by the 11th century. These stones relied on a similar principle to Seneca's bowl of water. A reading stone was simply a hemisphere of glass placed on top of the words to magnify the letters.

At that time the only people capable of making transparent glass were the glass blowers of Venice, so it is likely that the first spectacles were developed in Italy. One of the earliest inventors was probably the Dominican monk Alessandro da Spina from Florence around 1284, but there is no definite evidence for this.

The first mention of actual glasses is found in a 1289 manuscript, when a member of the Florentine Popozo family wrote in a manuscript entitled *Traite de con uite de la famille, di Popozo*:

> *I am so debilitated by age that without the glasses known as spectacles, I would no longer be able to read or write. These have recently been invented for the benefit of poor old people whose sight has become weak.*

The first designs didn't have sides and had to be held on the nose. Poorer people had theirs mounted in leather, wood, horn, bone or even light steel, while the upper classes had gold or silver frames.

For centuries, nobody found a good way to hold spectacles in place. Spanish spectacle makers tied silk ribbons on to the frames, which could be looped over the ears, and the Chinese added little weights to the end of the ribbons. It was only in 1730 that an English instrument maker, Edward Scarlett, designed spectacles with rigid side arms.

Valves in Veins

Hieronymus Fabricius ab Aquapendente (1537–1619)

When Fabricius discovered that veins had valves, his work provided the basis upon which his student William Harvey later described the circulation of the blood – often quoted as one of the most influential discoveries in medical history.

When Fabricius was alive, it was widely accepted that the body had blood in the veins and that there was a completely separate supply of blood in the arteries. This idea was based on the theories of Claudius Galen (129–216 AD), a 2nd-century physician who believed that the arteries were the source of vitality and the veins carried the source of nourishment and growth. In his view, blood was made in the liver and attracted to the different organs when the organs needed nourishment.

Fabricius was an anatomist and embryologist working in Padua, Italy. He studied arteries and veins and made a thorough description of the valves in the veins, published in *De venarum ostiolis* in 1603, after demonstrating his theory in 1597 to his colleagues. He observed that there were only valves in the veins, and not in the arteries, except in the two large arteries at their origin from the heart. He believed (correctly) that their role was to stop the blood from pooling in the extremities, which would prevent central and upper parts from getting blood.

He had an international reputation, which attracted the English anatomist William Harvey (1578–1657) as his pupil between 1600–1602. Fabricius' work on the veins is significant because it was a building block in Harvey's subsequent theory of the circulation in 1628, which completely overtook Galenic theory.

Forceps

Peter Chamberlen (1560–1631)

*The forceps is a metal instrument designed to
ease a prolonged labour and deliver a healthy child.
Since its introduction it has saved the lives of
millions of women and babies.*

Although the mention of the word 'forceps' can strike fear into a pregnant woman, when used correctly, a forceps provides less pressure on the baby's head than the woman's birth canal.

The two blades of the instrument are inserted separately and cradle the baby's head, rather like two slim hands. The blades are then locked together in that position so that there is no way they can crush the baby's head. Then the baby is literally pulled out.

It was probably Peter Chamberlen who first used the instrument. He was the son of a French Huguenot who had fled France to escape persecution and settled in Southampton, England. Chamberlen's success in obstetrics led to his appointment as physician to King James I (1566–1625) of England (also James VI of Scotland) and his wife, Anne of Denmark (1574–1619).

However, when it was first introduced the forceps was kept a secret. Apparently when called to a birth, Chamberlen would hide the instrument in a box so that no-one saw it.

In the 17th century, when Chamberlen first used the forceps, inexperienced midwives with little medical knowledge attended most deliveries. Gradually these midwives were replaced with accoucheurs, or 'man-midwives'. They were doctors with some knowledge of anatomy and also some medical instruments. By 1730 accoucheurs were also beginning to use the Chamberlen forceps.

The original Chamberlen forceps were found in 1813 in a trunk in the attic of Woodham Mortimer Hall, near Maldon in Essex, home of the late Peter Chamberlen III (1601–1683), a descendant of the instrument's inventor.

One of the best-known accoucheurs was Scottish-born William Smellie (1697–1763), who was described as '*a great horse godmother of a he-midwife*' by midwife Elizabeth Nihell. Smellie was the first person to teach obstetrics and midwifery on a scientific basis. He wrote the book *Midwifery,* published in 1752, which provides us with the very first detailed description of the obstetric forceps; he also set down rules for how to use the forceps safely.

The Microscope

Zacharias Janssen (1580–1638)

Being able to magnify an object many hundreds of times has enabled scientists to discover details about the structure of the world around us and more about the inner workings of the body. In medicine today, the microscope is vital to the identification of diseases and infections.

The Romans discovered that if you looked at an object through a piece of glass that was thick in the middle and thin on the edges, it magnified the object. They called these pieces of glass '*lenses*', from the Latin word lentil, because they looked the same shape as a lentil bean. However, it wasn't until the end of the 13th century that spectacle makers started to use lenses to be worn as glasses.

It was a Dutch spectacle maker who was probably the first to discover that lenses could be used to make a microscope. In 1590, Zacharias Janssen (1580–1638) put several lenses in a tube and discovered that the object near the end of the tube appeared much bigger.

Most historians believe that Zacharias' father Hans was also involved in this discovery, as his son would have been very young at the time. Whoever is responsible, this was the first known compound microscope – using two lenses.

Word travelled, and many people were interested in the invention that began to be known as the 'microscope'. In Italy, physiologist and physician Marcello Malpighi (1628–1694) made a huge contribution to the popularity of the microscope when, in 1661, he discovered the network of capillaries that connect the small veins to the small arteries in the lungs. This discovery reinforced Harvey's theory of the circulation and

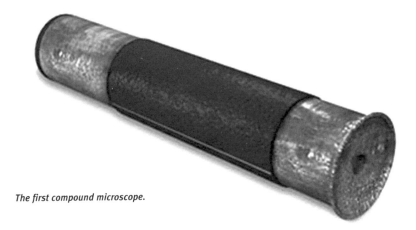

The first compound microscope.

finally overturned the previous view that blood was used up by the tissues.

Malpighi also wrote detailed descriptions of the anatomy of the tongue – including the first description of the taste buds, the skin, the brain, the liver and gall bladder and the heart.

In England, the scientist Robert Hooke (1635–1703) was among the first to make significant improvements to Janssen's original design, although it was actually Christopher Cock, a London-based instrument maker, who made the instruments.

Hooke used his microscope to make extensive studies of the world around him, publishing his findings in *Micrographia* in 1665. The book contains 38 beautifully hand drawn plates including investigations into lice, snow, a razor, a needle, and so on. In cork he saw pores, which he called 'cells' – the first description of cells in biology.

Inspired by Hooke's *Micrographia*, Dutchman Anthony van Leeuwenhoek (1632–1723), a draper from Delft, began to learn how to make his own lenses. He had previously been using a magnifying glass to count threads in woven cloth. By grinding and polishing, he was able to make small lenses with great curvatures. These rounder lenses produced greater magnification, and his microscopes were able to magnify up to 270 times. Although these microscopes were basically strong magnifying glasses using just one lens, their magnification exceeded the compound microscopes based on Janssen's original design that were available at the time.

In all, van Leeuwenhoek made many hundreds of microscopes. Even though he had no scientific background he made studies of wood, the cells of plants and the fine structure of animal bodies – he saw red blood corpuscles and blood capillaries and the crystals in gout. He confirmed Malpighi's findings about the circulation and he made detailed descriptions of nerves, muscles, bone, teeth and hair, 67 species of insect, 11 species of spider and 10 of crustacea.

Even though he didn't invent the microscope, van Leeuwenhoek is often described as one of the significant people in the discovery, as his microscope was so powerful and he made such significant discoveries with it.

See: *Harvey and the Circulation of Blood,* pages 29–30

Harvey and the Circulation of Blood

William Harvey (1578–1657)

*Harvey was the first to accurately describe
how the heart pumps the blood in a circular
course around the body, through the arteries,
into the veins and back to the heart.*

By carefully studying the flow of blood in living animals and by dissecting the bodies of animals and criminals, Harvey was able to formulate his theory of the human circulation which was published in his book *Exercitatio Anatomica de Motu Cordis et Sanguinis in Animalibus – An Anatomical Exercise Concerning the Motion of the Heart and Blood in Animals* (1628).

Before then most people believed that the body made new blood as it used up the old, and that there were two types of blood – in the veins and in the arteries.

This was based on the theories of Galen (129–216 AD), a 2nd-century physician, who believed that nourishment and growth came via the venous blood, which originated in the liver, while vitality originated in the heart and was carried in the arteries.

In 1600–1602 Harvey studied at the University of Padua where he was taught by Hieronymous Fabricius (1537–1619), before returning to work as a doctor at St Bartholomew's Hospital in London. It was Fabricius's discovery of valves in the veins that led to Harvey's theory of the circulation.

When Harvey's book was first published, very few of his colleagues believed it, partly because abandoning the accepted view in favour of the circulation of blood also called into question the widely trusted technique of blood letting – carried out in the belief that a fever resulted from too much blood in the body.

Although it took decades for Harvey's theories to be widely accepted, his work now underpins modern research into cardiovascular medicine and is widely considered to be one of the greatest medical breakthroughs.

See: *Valves in Veins,* page 23

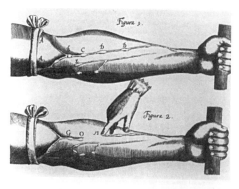

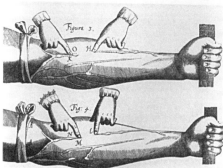

This illustration depicts one of William Harvey's experiments in his book **On the Circulation of the Blood** *(1628).*

The presence of valves in the veins had already been discovered. Harvey shows that blood in the veins flows towards the heart. He put a tournequet around the arm to show up the veins. Then he smoothed the blood away from the heart and showed that the vein remains empty because of the valve.

Vacuum Extraction

James Yonge (1647–1721)

*For many years childbirth was a dangerous experience.
If the baby didn't deliver easily, there weren't many
ways to assist the mother.*

Forceps were not invented until the late 16th century, and for over 100 years they were the secret of the Chamberlen family and so not widely used. Until the late 19th century, Caesarean sections were a last resort, to be used on a dying or dead woman to extract the baby. So it was a great relief to women when a less traumatic option was developed, which relied on literally sucking the baby out of the womb.

The first attempted vacuum extraction, also known as ventouse, was probably undertaken by the English surgeon James Yonge (1647–1721) in 1706, who recorded putting a cupping glass on the baby's head to create an artificial vacuum.

Cupping was a technique that had been

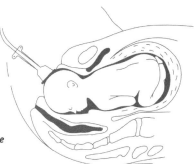

Attaching the suction cup to the baby's head helps to pull the baby out of its mother's womb.

used by healers in a number of different countries for centuries. It involved using a heated metal or glass cup over the area to be treated, such as a boil or a skin puncture. As the cup cooled, a vacuum developed in the cup, drawing blood or other fluids into it.Yonge's attempt to deliver the baby using this technique was unsuccessful, but it inspired others to adapt the idea. For example, James Simpson (1811–1870), a Scottish obstetrician, described a successful delivery with his Suction Tractor to the Edinburgh Obstetric Society in 1848.

However, the ventouse never really became popular until the 20th century, because more reliable methods for generating a vacuum were needed, as well as a better design for the cup.

After the Second World War (1939–1945), the vacuum extractor began to gain in popularity, as new technology was combined with the idea to produce several better designs. One of the best-known of these vacuum extractors was designed in 1952 by Viktor Finderle (1902–1964), a Croatian obstetrician. However, a stainless steel cup vacuum device introduced by Tage Malmström in Sweden in 1954, and modified by him in 1957, largely outmoded Finderle's version and is the antecedent of the modern models used today.

Current devices use more sophisticated technology to monitor and limit the pressure applied to the baby's head, which makes them safer to use.

See: *Forceps,* pages 24–25; *Caesarean Section,* pages 19–20

Prevention of Scurvy

James Lind (1716–1794)

Scurvy is due to a lack of dietary vitamin C, which can be found in fresh fruit and vegetables.

Although rare today, scurvy was very common among sailors in the 17th and 18th centuries, many of whom were at sea for months without access to fresh food. Whole crews could be decimated.

One of the worst episodes occurred in the 1740s, when Commodore George Anson (1697–1762) lost 1,300 out of 2,000 sailors on a voyage into the Pacific Ocean, most due to scurvy. Symptoms of scurvy included swollen, spongy, bleeding gums, huge bruises, swollen joints, exhaustion, heart failure and eventually death.

At the time there were many theories about the cause of scurvy, ranging from too much salt in the diet, to bad air and thickened blood. Various remedies were used to treat it, such as the boiled needles of the Eastern White Cedar (later found to contain high quantities of vitamin C), but nobody was certain of the best cure.

In 1734, Johann Bachstrom (1688–1742), a physician from Leiden in Germany, published a book in which he described scurvy as a disease '*owing to a total abstinence from fresh vegetable food, and greens*' and recommended fresh fruit and vegetables to treat it. However, it was James Lind (1716–1794) who first proved that scurvy could be treated and prevented by adding citrus fruit to the diet.

Lind was an Edinburgh surgeon serving on HMS *Salisbury* in 1747, when he carried out his research. He selected 12 men suffering from the disease and divided them into six pairs. He gave each pair a different addition to their basic diet. Some had seawater, others cider, one group had a mixture of garlic, mustard and horseradish. One group was given two oranges and lemons, and this pair made a rapid and complete recovery. He published his findings in 1753 in *A Treatise of the Scurvy*:

> *The most sudden and visible good effects were perceived from the use of the oranges and lemons; one of those who had taken them, being at the end of six days fit for duty. The other was the best recovered of any in his condition.*

However, Lind didn't realise that scurvy was due to a lack of vitamin C. He thought that it was caused by moist air, and that the disease occurred because of a blockage in the normal sweating mechanism. In his view, lemon juice worked as a detergent which divided up the toxic particles, so that they could escape through the blocked skin pores.

During the Napoleonic Wars (1799–1815), it became standard practice for the British Royal Navy to take fresh limes on board to prevent scurvy, which gave rise to the name 'limey' for a British sailor.

It wasn't until over a hundred years later that Vitamin C was finally identified, linking Lind's earlier discoveries with the deficiency disease.

False Teeth

Alexis Duchâteau (1714–1792)

With the discovery of resins and plastics, it is now possible to fill a gap in the teeth with a denture that functions, isn't painful and looks realistic.

In the 16th century English queen Elizabeth I (1533–1603) reportedly plugged the gaps in her teeth with pieces of cloth when she appeared in public. Poorer people were often completely toothless. And, although people have been making false teeth since at least 700 BC, it is only since the discovery of porcelain dentures in the 18th century that they have been a real option.

Before then dentures were made out of bone, wood or ivory – often from a hippopotamus or walrus – that rotted fast because they were not enamelled. Teeth were also pulled from corpses and reused, and poor people donated their own teeth in exchange for money. Generally these human teeth were of pretty poor quality, often rotting before they were removed.

For many years it was normal practice to pull teeth out of soldiers' mouths on the battlefield, and wartime provided a generous supply of what were known as 'Waterloo teeth'. Generally these were of slightly better quality than the normal supply of human teeth, because dead soldiers were usually young.

Rotting false teeth produced a horrible taste and foul breath. Fans became fashionable to cover up both the teeth and the smell and many people preferred to go toothless.

Duchâteau was a French apothecary and was the first to make dentures out of porcelain in order to produce a result that looked more like real teeth and would last longer.

Parisian dentist Nicolas Dubois de Chemant (1753–1824), who worked for Duchâteau, was the first to patent the design in 1776. In *A Dissertation on Artificial Teeth in General* he wrote that the invention was:

A composition for the purpose of making of artificial teeth either single, double or in rows or in complete sets and also springs for fastening or affixing the same in a more easy and effectual manner than any hitherto discovered. Said teeth may be made of any shade or colour, which they will retain for any length of time and will consequently more perfectly resemble the natural teeth.

Josiah Wedgewood (1730–1795), an English pottery designer, supplied most of the porcelain paste. However, porcelain teeth tended to chip and break and were too white to be realistic. It was also hard to get a good fit in the mouth. As a result, artificial teeth did not become popular until around 1826, some 50 years later, after the discovery of vulcanized rubber made it possible to make better moulds and, therefore, properly fitting dentures. Subsequent advances in plastics and resins led to the manufacture of teeth that were more natural looking.

The Ambulance

Dominique Jean Larrey (1766–1842)

The idea of an ambulance that brings aid to an injured or sick patient originated on 11th-century battlefields.

The ambulance service has developed extensively so that now highly trained ambulance staff can provide life-saving treatment within minutes and transport a patient by air, road, sea or train to the nearest hospital.

The first-known first aiders were the Knights of St John. They treated soldiers on the battlefield during the Crusades in the 11th century. The practice of moving injured soldiers off the battlefield developed in the 15th century, when the Spanish army used *ambulancarias*, or military hospitals, for the first time.

The first official ambulances were created by Baron Dominique Larrey (1766–1842), the Surgeon-in-Chief of the French Grand Army, and used by Napoleon's (1769–1821) army in 1793. Larrey's *ambulances volantes* were horse-drawn wagons used to transport trained attendants to give first aid on the battlefield and then carry them back with the injured soldiers to the field hospitals.

The first ambulance based at a civilian hospital was in 1865 at Commercial Hospital, Cincinnati in the United States. This was soon followed by others, notably the New York service provided out of Bellevue Hospital. These hospital ambulances were left harnessed to the horses so that they could move quickly, and carried medical supplies.

The first motor-powered ambulance (1899) followed the introduction of the motorcar. Since then, with research into the value of early treatment, ambulances have become further specialized, with the introduction of air ambulances and cardiac ambulances with crew, trained to administer life-saving drugs at the scene.

Smallpox Vaccine

Edward Jenner (1749–1823)

In 1977 Smallpox became the first disease to be completely eradicated from the world as a result of a successful vaccination programme.

In the late 18th century, Edward Jenner was working as an English country doctor. Smallpox was rife – as many as one in ten people were affected – and it was usually fatal.

Jenner noticed that milkmaids who were infected with cowpox – a disease of cattle that occasionally affected humans – were protected against smallpox. Cowpox in humans is a mild disease, so Jenner thought perhaps there might be a safe way of using this knowledge to protect people against smallpox.

In 1796 he removed a small amount of the discharge inside a milkmaid's cowpox pustule and injected it into an eight-year-old boy. Although he developed a fever, he soon recovered. Six weeks later Jenner injected the discharge from a smallpox pustule into the same boy, and nothing happened. The boy was protected from smallpox by the cowpox vaccine. Jenner's results quickly caught on – and by 1799 over 5,000 people had been vaccinated.

See: *The Eradication of Smallpox,* page 141

Colour Blindness

John Dalton (1766–1844)

Colour blindness is when the eye doesn't recognize certain colours in the spectrum – most commonly red and green.

Colour blindness is the result of a problem in the specialized cells called cones, found in the light-sensitive lining at the back of the eye, or retina.

John Dalton, who first described colour blindness, was a chemist and physicist interested in many things besides vision. Notably, he was the first person to develop atomic theory, and he also found time to write detailed accounts of the weather every day for over 50 years.

He and his brother were both colour blind, inspiring him to investigate the problem in more detail. In his paper *Extraordinary Facts Relating To the Vision of Colours* he wrote:

That part of the image which others call red appears to me little more than a shade or defect of light. After

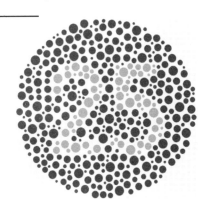

This is an example of an Ishihara plate. The dots that comprise the number '25' are red; the surrounds green. Someone with red–green colour blindness would not be able to see anything except a series of grey dots. People with normal colour vision see the number.

that the orange, yellow and green seem one colour which descends pretty uniformly from an intense to a rare yellow, making what I should call different shades of yellow.

Dalton's preserved eyeball was examined in 1995 and found to have red–green colour blindness, but there are many other types. It is usually an inherited condition, and one that primarily affects men.

Because of his contribution to the field, the condition of colour blindness is sometimes called Daltonism.

For years, it was difficult to diagnose colour blindness. In 1916, the Japanese ophthalmologist Shinobu Ishihara (1879–1963) devised a system for testing for colour blindness in soldiers. His testing system is still used today and is known as the Ishihara plates. These are a series of coloured numbers with coloured backgrounds (*see illustration*).

Women Medical Students

Miranda Stuart (1795–1865)

Until quite recently, there was considerable prejudice against allowing women entry to medical school. Determined that she was going to succeed in her wish to train as a doctor, Miranda Stewart resorted to dressing up as a man in order to gain a place.

Miranda Stuart enrolled in the University of Edinburgh's medical school in 1809, 36 years before Elizabeth Blackwell (1821–1910) got a place to study medicine in America.

Stuart (aka James Barry) qualified in 1812 and became an Army Surgeon in 1819, where she rose to the most senior rank of Medical Inspector. Although she was criticized by Lord Albermale for '*a certain effeminacy*' in her manner, she kept the pretence going until her death, when her secret was uncovered.

Women have not always had so much difficulty in gaining acceptance in medicine. In Ancient Egypt there were many female students and doctors, but gradually it became less acceptable, and by the Middle Ages it was not possible. In fact, in 1421 a petition was presented to the English king Henry V (1387–1422) to prevent women from practising medicine – the historical equivalent of protecting jobs for the boys. Women continued to work as midwives until the 19th century, when men took over that role too with the emergence of obstetrics and gynaecology as a specialism.

Elizabeth Blackwell was the first woman to be accepted to medical school without pretending to be a man. She was born in England but moved to the United States as a small child. She became a teacher in a school set up by her mother after her father died, but she found it boring and uninspiring. Once she had decided to train as a doctor she applied to more than 15 medical schools before being accepted at a small one in Geneva, New York. Despite being ostracized and harassed by her fellow students, she qualified in 1849, with top marks in her class.

In the United Kingdom, the first group of women medical students were known as the Edinburgh Seven. They campaigned long and hard to be allowed to study medicine at the University of Edinburgh and they won in 1869, when they were allowed to attend. However, a legal challenge in 1873 meant that they were not awarded their degrees.

Over time, women-only medical schools were opened. However, doctors who qualified here found it hard to get employment anywhere except in one of these schools. Prejudice was still entrenched, and many men had strong views on the subject. In 1905 the President of the Oregon State Medical Society, Dr Van Dyk, wrote that educated women *'could not bear children with ease because study arrested the development of the pelvis'*.

Even when women were eventually allowed to enter medical schools the opposition continued, with comments that women doctors were *'emotionally unstable'*, *'talked too much'* and *'got pregnant'*. A dean of one school claimed he would prefer a *'third-rate man to a first-rate woman doctor'*.

Things have moved on gradually, and although the percentage of women in medical schools was still only about six per cent in 1950, it has risen steadily. In the United Kingdom the proportion of women medical students exceeded 50 per cent in 1991, and has continued to rise ever since.

The Stethoscope

René-Théophile-Hyacinthe Laënnec (1781–1826)

*Laënnec's invention marked the beginning of a
new era in the ability to diagnose disease.*

Until the 19th century doctors had to rely on the description of symptoms given by the patient and examination of the external body alone. The stethoscope enabled doctors to get more objective information about the internal body.

Laënnec was a highly respected French doctor who at the time of his discovery was chief of the Necker Hospital in Paris. He first wrote about the concept of the stethoscope and how he used it to examine a young woman consulting him with symptoms of heart disease in 1816:

I recalled a well-known acoustic phenomenon: namely, if you place your ear against one end of a wooden beam, the scratch of a pin at the other extremity is distinctly audible. It occurred to me that this physical property might serve a useful purpose in the case with which I was then dealing. Taking a sheet of paper I rolled it into a very tight roll, one end of which I placed on the precordial region, whilst I put my ear to the other. I was both surprised and gratified at being able to hear the beating of the heart with much greater clearness and distinctness than I had ever before by direct application of my ear.

The first stethoscope was made of wood and for one ear only. It was 23cm/9in. long and 4cm/1½ in. in diameter, made out of two pieces screwed together with detachable ear and chest pieces. Using this instrument it was possible to distinguish between different types of breath and heart sounds. Doctors were now able to accurately diagnose conditions such as pneumonia and tuberculosis.

Later modifications to Laënnec's invention included rubber tubing. In 1852 George Cammann (1804–1863), an American doctor, created the stethoscope that any patient would recognize today.

Laënnec published details of his discovery in 1819, in his *Traité de l'Auscultation Médiate*. News of the discovery spread fast, incorporated even in *Middlemarch* (1871–1872) by celebrated English novelist George Eliot (pseudonym of Mary Anne Evans, 1819–1880). In the book Tertius Lydgate, just back from his medical training in Paris, describes the new invention to sceptical older colleagues.

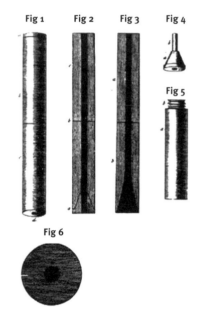

Laennec's stethoscope from De l'Auscultation Mediate *(1819).*
Figure (1) Instrument assembled
Figures (2) & (3) Two forms of the instrument in longitudinal section
Figure (4) Detachable chest piece
Figure (5) Ear piece unscrewed
Figure (6) Transverse section

Intravenous Fluids

Thomas Aitchison Latta (c. 1790–1833)

During the cholera epidemic of 1831–1832, Latta was the first to realize that patients were dying of dehydration and that intravenous treatment could help.

Latta wrote about his findings in a letter to the medical journal *The Lancet*, describing how he had infused six pints of fluid into an elderly patient with cholera who was near death.

He described how:

soon the sharpened features, and sunken eye, and fallen jaw, pale and cold, bearing the manifest imprint of death's signet, began to glow with returning animation; the pulse returned to the wrist... Thirty minutes later the woman announced that she was free from all uneasiness.

Latta's prescription was for '*two drachmas of muriate, two scruples of carbonative soda and 60 ounces of water*', otherwise known as a primitive solution of saline, or salty water, similar, in fact, to what is used today.

Latta's treatment was based on the findings of another physician Dr William O'Shaughnessy (1808–1889), a graduate from the University of Edinburgh who, earlier in the same year, had been sent to Newcastle by the Royal College of Surgeons in London to study the blood of cholera patients. O'Shaughnessy found that there was:

a great but variable deficiency of water in the blood in four malignant cholera cases; a total absence of carbonate of soda in two; and a remarkable diminution of the other saline ingredients.

O'Shaughnessy's conclusion was that the only way to help these patients was to inject fluid into their veins.

Latta's infusion method gained some followers, notably Dr John MacKintosh, based at the Drummond Street Cholera Hospital in Edinburgh. The treatment was reserved for patients near death, and who would otherwise definitely die. MacKintosh found that of 156 patients who received the intravenous fluid, 25 recovered.

However, the advances made in this method of treatment ceased once the cholera epidemic ended, simply because there was less need or opportunity to continue studying the disease or its treatment. Latta died the following year of tuberculosis and O'Shaughnessy left for India the same year. By the time the next cholera epidemic came to Edinburgh a decade later, in 1848–1849, many doctors had forgotten about intravenous fluids. Detailed records show that of the 739 cholera victims, only 27 were given intravenous saline while 78 had blood drained through venesection. Intravenous fluid treatment took another 75 years to become widely accepted within the medical community.

Beaumont's Experiments on the Gastric Juice

William Beaumont (1785–1853)

The liquid produced by the stomach is an acid and digestion is a chemical process.

Beaumont's work challenged the previously held view that the fluid found in the stomach was like water.

William Beaumont was a surgeon working in the United States army in the 19th century. In 1822 he looked after a young man who had been shot in the stomach, leaving a gaping wound. Beaumont covered the wound with a metal plate and, although the hole never healed, the man recovered sufficiently to marry and to have four children of his own.

In the years that followed, Beaumont conducted many experiments on his patient to investigate the appearance and properties of the digestive fluid. He introduced various bits of food tied to a silk string into the stomach via the hole, and then retrieving them to see the effects. As a result of these observations, he concluded that the digestive process was a chemical process of dissolving the food, rather than squashing or macerating it.

Beaumont's work was published in 1833 in *Experiments and Observations on the Gastric Juice and the Physiology of Digestion*, which made him famous.

General Anaesthetic

William E. Clarke (1818–1878)

Before the discovery of general anaesthetics, patients endured unimaginable agony in surgery.

Until the 1840s patients often had to be held down by several assistants before they passed out. Many died on the table during surgery, while those that survived were severely traumatized by the experience.

Charles Darwin (1809–1882) commented on this in his autobiography:

I also attended on two occasions the operating theatre in the hospital at Edinburgh, and saw two very bad operations, one on a child, but I rushed away before they were completed. Nor did I ever attend again, for hardly any inducement would have been strong enough to make me do so; this being long before the blessed days of chloroform. The two cases fairly haunted me for many a long year.

For centuries doctors had used opium and alcohol to try to reduce the pain of surgery. Other treatments included hyoscyamine, which was similar to opium, and mandrake, which was famously used to send Juliet into a reversible coma in William Shakespeare's (1564–1616) play *Romeo and Juliet*. But none could completely dull the pain and surgery remained an excruciating and dangerous last resort.

Things began to change in 1795 when the British chemist Humphrey Davy (1778–1829) discovered that nitrous oxide, when mixed with oxygen, could produce pain relief and reversible unconsciousness. Although Davy realized the implications of his discovery for surgery, his theory was not tested until years later, when it began to be used more widely as pain relief during labour in the 20th century. Nitrous oxide was known as 'laughing gas', because inhaling it made people giggly and relaxed, making it more popular in funfairs than in doctors' surgeries.

In the 1840s, American doctors and dentists started using ether to anaesthetize patients before extracting their teeth. Ether had been discovered in 1275 by Spanish chemist Raymundus Lullius (c.1232–1315), and was originally called 'sweet oil of vitriol' before being renamed ether in 1730. The first to use it was William E. Clarke (1818–1878), a chemist and doctor from New York. He carried out a tooth extraction in 1842 using ether and his success inspired Crawford Long (1815–1878), a country doctor in Georgia, to remove a neck cyst using ether the same year.

Confidence grew, and the news of ether's success spread to Europe. Rapidly it became standard practice to anaesthetize the patient with ether prior to surgery.

However, ether tended to make patients cough and vomit. In the United Kingdom it was soon replaced by chloroform, which had first been discovered in 1831, but only grew in popularity as an anaesthetic in the late 1840s. In 1853 the British queen Victoria (1819–1901) used chloroform during the birth of her son Prince Leopold (1853–1884). She records in her journal that: *The effect was soothing, quieting and delightful beyond measure.*

The Vaginal Speculum

James Marion Sims (1813–1883)

In modern medical practice, the vaginal speculum is indispensable for examining the vagina and cervix.

———

In the past, if a woman survived the experience of giving birth, she was lucky if she escaped suffering from the damage caused to the tissues around the birth canal for several years. Many women became incontinent of urine and sometimes of faeces, too; in some cases, the supporting muscles and ligaments became so badly stretched or torn during childbirth that the uterus slipped down into the vagina as a result of gravity, causing a prolapse.

Women were often too ashamed or embarrassed to seek help in such cases. It was considered improper to examine a woman's genitals and so intimate examinations were not routine. As a result, doctors had limited experience at diagnosis in these areas.

The tools available for examining women internally were primitive and most doctors relied on touch to make a diagnosis. Although speculums have been in existence since ancient times, it was not until the 18th century that interest grew in improving the equipment used for more detailed examination of women.

One surgeon who was keen to help these women was James Sims (1813–1883), a general practitioner from Alabama, United States whose first speculum was fashioned out of a pewter spoon, which held the vaginal walls open so it was possible to examine the birth canal. Known as the Sims Speculum, the resulting prototype has gone on to inspire one of the most widely used instruments, and is still in use today.

Sims has been lauded and criticized with equal measure. He has been called the Father of Gynaecology in the United

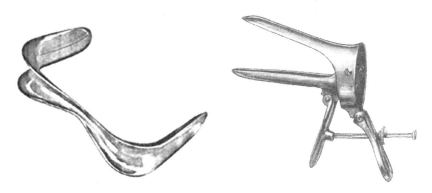

The first bivalved speculum was introduced in 1801 by Joseph Claude Recamier (1774–1852). Numerous modifications were made on Recamier's original design, including the Sims speculum (left), a simpler form of the more popular speculum in use today (right).

States and his statue graces New York's Central Park. At the same time, though, Sims has been criticized because a lot of his work in helping women damaged in childbirth was the result of repeated experimental surgery he carried out without anaesthesia on three black slave women. Once he had perfected his surgical techniques, he carried out surgery on white women suffering from the damage caused by childbirth – but with these women he used anaesthetic.

Spirometry

John Hutchinson (1811–1861)

A spirometer measures how well the lung functions and is used to assess and monitor lung disease.

Scientists have always been fascinated with measuring respiration. The first documented experiments were carried out in the 2nd century, when the influential physician Galen (AD 129–216) found that if a boy breathed in and out of a dead animal's bladder, the volume of the gas did not change. It was not until 14 centuries later that the famous mathematician and physicist Giovanni Borelli (1608–1679) became the first person to try to measure this volume by sucking a liquid into a cylinder after blocking his nostrils.

In the 18th and 19th centuries, scientists continued conducting experiments. One experient involved putting a man in a hogshead up to his chin, and measuring the rise and fall in the level of the water in the cylinder as he breathed!

However, in 1844 there was a significant development, when English surgeon John Hutchinson (1811–1861) published a paper

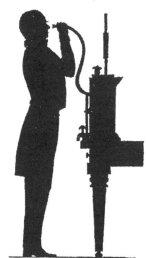

A silhouette of John Hutchinson and his spirometer, illustrating correct body positioning for performance of the vital capacity.

describing his water spirometer – a calibrated bell, inverted in water.

Hutchinson believed that the amount of air that could be exhaled after a full in-breath was an indicator of the health of the patient. People with a low measurement seemed to have a lower life expectancy. He called this the vital capacity – literally the capacity to live. Hutchinson lived at a time when tuberculosis (TB) was common and he believed that lung complications reduced the vital capacity and resulted in an early death. He studied over 2,000 patients who he grouped into:

Paupers
First Battalion Grenadier Guards
Pugilists and Wrestlers
Giants and Dwarfs
Girls
Gentleman
Deceased Cases

With the dead patients, he inserted a tube into the airway soon after death and then closed it so that no air could escape. Then he inflated the corpse using a bellows until no more air would go in. Then he released the valve in the airway, and measured the air that came out.

His detailed observations showed that the vital capacity was directly related to height – the taller you are, the bigger the vital capacity. With age, he found that the older you are, the lower the vital capacity, and vice versa.

Hutchinson claimed his instrument could detect lung disease earlier than listening to the patient with a stethoscope, and it didn't take an expert to interpret the results of the test.

Although few doctors used the spirometer in the 19th century, spirometry is now considered to be a useful way of predicting and diagnosing lung disease. The machines are smaller, and portable, providing more detailed measurements, but the principles are the same.

Hutchinson became a consultant to the insurance industry based in London, believing that the vital capacity should be used in actuarial predictions for people selling life insurance. He left England in a shroud of mystery on a ship bound for Australia leaving his wife and children behind. Some say it was because he had tuberculosis and the fresh air and rest was supposed to help him. He was found dead later in Fiji, aged just 50. Some people believe that Hutchinson was murdered.

Appendicectomy

Henry Hancock (1809–1880)

An operation to remove the appendix in modern times is a minor procedure, leaving minimal scarring and rarely requiring more than a few days rest in hospital for the patient. However, this has not always been the case.

Although appendicitis was first described in the 16th century, having been identified during post mortem examinations, it was not until two centuries later that doctors learnt how to correctly diagnose it in a living patient. Remedies have varied, from treatment with leeches, bloodletting and enemas to constant horseback riding or laying a newly killed and cut-open puppy across the patient! Not surprisingly, patients in such cases usually died.

The first description of the removal of an appendix was one done almost by accident when Claudius Amyand (c.1680–1740), surgeon and founder of St George's Hospital in London, removed it during the course of an operation for a hernia on an 11-year-old boy in 1735.

The first operation done specifically to remove the appendix is credited to Henry Hancock in 1848. He was a former president of the Royal Society of Medicine and was working as a surgeon in London when he was asked to attend to a 30-year-old woman with appendicitis.

Following his successful treatment and the patient's recovery, Hancock recommended surgical treatment for all cases at an early stage in the condition. Given the dangers of surgery at that time, Hancock's approach was considered cavalier by his contemporaries. However, he was proved right, and early removal is now considered most likely to have a successful outcome.

Ophthalmoscope

Hermann Ludwig Ferdinand von Helmholtz (1821–1894)

*The back of the eye is the only place in the body where
it is possible to examine the blood vessels closely.
Not only does this examination give information about
the state of the eye's health, but by inference,
it also informs doctors about the state of the blood
vessels in the rest of the body.*

Von Helmholtz wanted to study physics at university, but his family could not afford the fees. Instead he studied medicine, which was subsidized by the state, in return for a period of time working for the military. However, soon after he qualified it became clear that he was a talented scientist, and he was released early from his military commitments to pursue a career in academic science. He became professor at the University of Konigsberg, teaching physiology (the study of the body's functions). Over the next 22 years he moved to the universities at Bonn and Heidelberg, and it was during this time that he conducted his most significant work in medicine.

Among other things, Helmholtz began to study the human eye. Little was known at the time about what lay beyond the pupil.

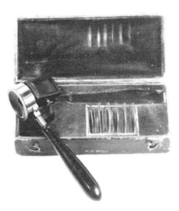

The opthalmoscope, originally pioneered by Herman von Helmholtz in the 19th century.

After only a few months, he had designed and built his first ophthalmoscope out of cardboard, glue and microscope glass plates, and called it the *Augenspiegel* (eye mirror). The name ophthalmoscope (eye-observer) was introduced in 1854.

Helmholtz's instrument consisted of three plates of glass pressed together and mounted on a handle at a 45° angle. A light source – in his case this was a candle – was placed beside the patient. Some light passed through the plates but some was reflected back into the eye.

Since Helmholtz's invention, ophthalmoscopes have become more sophisticated, with electric light sources inside them, and focusing lenses to allow examination of the eye at different depths and magnifications, but the basic principle remains unchanged.

In recognition of his contribution to the study of physiology and optics, Helmholtz received the inheritable suffix 'von' from Kaiser Wilhelm I in 1882.

See: *Spectacles,* pages 21–22

Plaster of Paris Casts

Antonius Mathijsen (1805–1878)

Nikolai Ivanovich Pirogov (1810–1881)

*Casts made from Plaster of Paris replaced more
traditional splints in the mid 19th century.*

Plaster of Paris is calcium sulphate hemi-hydrate ($CaSO_4 0.5H_2O$) derived from gypsum – a sedimentary rock consisting of calcium sulphate dihydrate ($CaSO_4 2H_2O$). It is produced when gypsum is fired at relatively low temperature and then reduced to powder.

When water is added to Plaster of Paris, the calcium sulphate hemi-hydrate returns to the relatively insoluble calcium sulphate dihydrate (gypsum) and also produces heat. It takes about 10 minutes for the plaster to set.

After a bone breaks, it has to be realigned first with a splint and then held in place with some kind of rigid plaster. The idea of using stiffened bandages to hold a fracture in position wasn't new and previously doctors had used anything from waxes and resins to lime derived from sea shells, or animal fat, egg and flour mixtures to have the same effect as Plaster of Paris.

Antonius Mathijsen, a Flemish military surgeon, was the first to use bandages impregnated with Plaster of Paris to combine the features of a splint and a bandage in the treatment of fractures. He wrote an account of this treatment in 1852. By wetting the bandages and then wrapping them around the limb that needed to be kept in a particular position, Mathijsen showed that it was possible to create a perfectly fitting rigid splint to hold the bones in place without any assistance.

At the same time, Nikolai Ivanovich Pirogov, Professor of Surgery at the Academy of Military Medicine in St Petersburg, Russia, introduced the use of Plaster of Paris dressing in the treatment of casualties in the Crimean War (1853–1856). Pirogov was aware of Mathijsen's work, but his method was to soak coarse cloth in a Plaster of Paris mixture immediately before applying it.

Mathijsen's method became more widely used, and for a long time the impregnated bandages were made by nurses. It wasn't until 1931 that these bandages were produced commercially

The use of Plaster of Paris casts was standard practice in the treatment of fractures, until the 1990s, when they started to be replaced by lighter, resin-based casts.

The Hypodermic Syringe

Charles Gabriel Pravaz (1791–1853)
Alexander Wood (1817–1884)

An astounding medical breakthrough, the hypodermic syringe has helped save lots of lives, but has also been used over the centuries by billions of drug addicts.

Although medicines had been applied to the skin for centuries, the invention of the hypodermic syringe allowed treatment to be administered directly in the person's veins. This led later to the development of the first general anaesthetic.

Credit for the invention of the hypodermic syringe is usually shared between two doctors. The first was a french doctor called Charles Gabriel Pravaz, who is also credited with being the first to understand the principles of how to treat congenital dislocation of the hip, and spent most of his life studying curvature of the spine. He was working in Lyon, France, when he made a syringe out of silver attached to a fine hollow needle. His invention gained wide acceptance and was known as 'The Pravaz Syringe'. It was first used to inject morphine as a painkiller.

At around the same time, the Scottish physician Alexander Wood, working in Edinburgh, had been experimenting with a hollow needle for the administration of drugs. Wood didn't invent the syringe and hollow needle but modified a design already manufactured by a local chemist – a Mr Ferguson of Giltspur Street, London. Wood published his findings in *The Edinburgh Medical and Surgical Review*, showing in his paper that the method was not necessarily limited to the administration of opiates, although ironically Wood's wife died from an overdose of injected morphine.

Although these two doctors are credited with the invention, in fact the knowledge of how to inject into a vein was not new. Almost two centuries earlier, in 1659, Sir Christopher Wren (1632–1723), the English architect who designed St Paul's Cathedral in London, became the first person to inject liquid into a vein.

Various doctors had subsequently experimented with Wren's technique, including the Irish surgeon Francis Rynd (1803–1861), who in 1845, developed a special instrument, that could inject a morphine solution beneath the skin. However, Rynd did not write down a description of his invention until 1861.

Sanitation

John Snow (1813–1858)

Before the discovery of a link between germs and disease, drinking water pumps were often contaminated with infected sewage, which led to the spread of disease.

In the 1830s, cholera was rampant across Europe, and the death rate was alarmingly high. At the time, the theory was that diseases were the result of gases produced by rotting and decomposing food and other organic matter. But when John Snow, a London doctor, questioned this theory, it resulted in one of the biggest medical breakthroughs of all.

In 1849 over 50,000 people died of cholera in England. Instead of the disease being spread by gases, as was believed by some experts, John Snow believed it was spread by infected diarrhoea seeping into the wells or rivers and contaminating the drinking water.

Five years later, in 1854, during an outbreak of cholera among the local

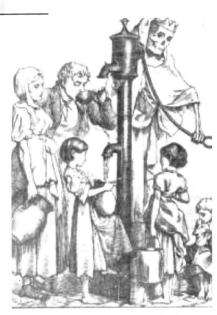

Death dispensing infected water to hapless victims, from a cartoon originally published in Fun *magazine, 1866.*

P Pump
- Cholera death
- Contanminated pump

A 19th-century map of London's Soho showing cholera cases around the Broad St water pump.

communities in Soho, London where Snow was working at the time, he collected detailed information about each case and discovered that nearly all the victims had used water from one water pump in Broad Street. Suspecting that this pump was contaminated with infected sewage, Snow requested the removal of the handle, which promptly stopped the outbreak and confirmed his theory.

Snow's discovery that cholera was spread by water and not by air had a great influence on health. Deaths from diarrhoea and dysentery fell steadily, with the poorest communities experiencing the greatest improvements in health. Today, experts believe that the provision of clean water and hygienic sanitation remains the main priority in bringing about an improvement in world health. Snow's contribution to medicine is widely believed to have had a bigger impact than any drug or surgical procedure since.

See: *Intravenous Fluids*, pages 45–46.

Nursing

Florence Nightingale (1820–1910)
Mary Seacole (1805–1881)

Although nurses had been in existence for centuries, these two women were the first to firmly establish that there was a key role for nurses in treating the sick.

Florence Nightingale helped establish nursing as an acceptable professional vocation for women – first in London, and consequently all over the world.

In Catholic countries such as France, nurses were traditionally members of religious orders, such as the Daughters of Charity set up in 1633 by Vincent de Paul (1581–1660) and Louise de Marillac (1591–1660). The sisters provided practical nursing skills, including the application of drugs and undertaking simple surgical procedures. Nuns were sent to train in Paris with the Daughters of Charity from Ireland, and then sent to other parts of the empire to Catholic communities.

Similar enterprises sprung up among protestants, notably the Deaconess Institute, established in 1836 by Theodore Fliedner (1800–1864) and his wife Friederike (1800–1842) in Kaiserswerth near Dusseldorf.

After much protest from her well-connected family, Florence Nightingale trained in both Kaiserswerth and with the Daughters of Charity in Paris. When the Crimean War (1853–1856) broke out, reports of the dreadful hospital conditions inspired her to take action. She persuaded her friend, Sidney Herbert (1810–1861), head of the War Office in London, to let her take a group of 38 nurses to the front line in Constantinople (then part of the Ottoman Empire, now part of present–day Turkey). This was the first time that female nurses had served in wartime field hospitals, and was a major achievement. There Nightingale found about 2,000 wounded and sick, and many more arrived daily. She believed that infection arose spontaneously in dirty and poorly ventilated environments, and she encouraged her nurses to combine a caring approach with a strict enforcement of cleanliness.

Initially the death toll rose. After six months, a sanitary commission was sent to Scutari (now a suburb of Istanbul, Turkey). They organized for the sewers to be flushed out and the ventilation improved. Death rates fell sharply after this.

Nightingale continued to believe that disease was related to inadequate nutrition and exhaustion. However, with more experience her opinion shifted, and she eventually realized that most deaths were due to poor sanitation. This knowledge influenced Nightingale's later career and led to her campaign for strict sanitary conditions in hospitals.

Using her *Notes on Nursing*, published in 1859, as the basis for training nurses in theory and practice, Florence Nightingale went on to set up a nursing school at St Thomas' Hospital, London, in 1860 on her return to the United Kingdom. Graduates from her nursing school also helped to set up nurses' training institutes in Sweden and Australia in 1867, the United States in 1873, Canada in 1874 and Denmark in 1897.

Mary Seacole is the less well known of the two nursing pioneers of the 19th century, but she was equally influential in the birth of, and giving credence to, the nursing profession. She was born in Jamaica and married a descendant of Horatio Nelson (1758–1805), travelling with him widely before he died. In her 50s, she became concerned about the welfare of soldiers in the Crimean War and travelled to Britain to offer her help as a nursing volunteer to Florence Nightingale.

She was rejected, but travelled to the Crimea anyway, setting up the British Hotel at her own cost to provide nourishment and nursing care to soldiers just a couple of miles from where the fighting was taking place. Seacole's main achievement was in recognizing the importance of providing nursing care on the battlefield, which was vital, particularly as the British military hospitals at which Florence Nightingale and her nurses worked were three days' sailing away from the front.

See: *Sanitation*, page 61–62.

The Treatment of Epilepsy

Sir Charles Locock (1799–1875)

Locock was the first person to recommend an effective medication for epilepsy, ending centuries of myth and superstition about causes and treatment for this distressing condition.

There have been many beliefs about the causes of epilepsy. Some people thought it was the result of phlegm blocking the airways, causing convulsions in the body as it tried to escape. Others believed it was due to angry gods or overzealous masturbation. It wasn't until the 17th century that people began to realize that epilepsy was actually a brain disorder.

Along with the range of beliefs, there have been as many and varied treatments. In the 6th century, Greek physician Alexander of Tralles (525–605) said that epileptics should:

take the nail of a wrecked ship, make it into a bracelet and set therein the bone of a stag's heart taken from its body whilst alive; put it on the left arm, and you will be astonished at the result,

In the 13th century, John of Gaddesden (c.1280–1361), the physician to English king Edward II (1284–1327) claimed success with his treatment which involved the patient wearing peony and chrysanthemum amulets or being covered in the hair of a white dog while he recited the Gospels.

Mistletoe has been used widely as a folk cure for epilepsy. In the 17th century, Robert Boyle (1627–1691), a leading figure in the development of chemistry, advocated that the patient should carry:

as much pulverized mistletoe as can be held on a six pence coin, early in the morning, in black cherry juice, during several days around the full moon.

The perception of epilepsy began to shift when famous anatomist Thomas Willis (1621–1675) wrote *Cerebri Anatome* (*Anatomy of the Brain*) in 1664. His work was based on detailed dissection, vivisection and clinical experience. Together with Willis' s book *Pathologiae cerebri et nervosi generis specimen* (*Pathology of the Brain, and Specimen of the Nature of the Nerves*) published in 1667, he influenced others to develop the idea that epilepsy might be a treatable disorder of the brain.

Gradually, epileptic patients were seen differently. Previously, many had been incarcerated in asylums for the insane, but by the mid-19th century special hospitals for epileptics had been established in France, Britain and Germany.

Sir Charles Locock, who was physician to Queen Victoria (1819–1901), and delivered all five of her children, was the first to recognize the anticonvulsant properties of potassium bromide. Although it had side effects, it was the only drug treatment available for nearly 60 years and marked a significant shift for the treatment of epilepsy away from witchcraft and folklore.

Mendel and the Birth of Genetics

Gregor Mendel (1822–1884)

Although the idea that certain family characteristics – such as the colour of eyes or hair – could be passed down through generations had been discussed for some time, there was much debate about how this actually happened until, that is, a 19th-century Austrian monk began to conduct experiments crossbreeding peas. His revolutionary discoveries form the basis of genetics and heredity today.

G regor Mendel conducted a series of experiments using garden peas growing in the Augustinian monastery in Brno in Bohemia where he lived as one of the monks. He wanted to find the result of cross-breeding on seven pairs of characteristics: seed shape and colour, pod shape and colour, flower colour and position of flower, and lastly, stem length.

Mendel's work took seven years to conduct and his results have influenced generations of geneticists to come.

He noticed that characteristics were passed from generation to generation. So, for example, plants with green peas had offspring with green peas too. He realised as a result of his observations that some factors were more 'dominant', and others were not. Mendel called these 'dominant' and 'recessive' factors. We now refer to these factors as 'genes'.

Although Mendel reported his results in 1865, it was not until nearly 20 years later that his work was first taken seriously by scientists. Today he is often called the 'Father of Genetics'.

The Germ Theory of Disease

Joseph Lister (1827–1912)

*The idea that diseases were caused by germs
was a breakthrough in medicine.*

In the early 19th century the death rate after an operation was high, with most people dying from wound infections. At the time, people believed that harmful gases produced by rotting flesh caused disease. However, Joseph Lister, a surgeon working in Glasgow, had ideas that would challenge this theory.

Lister had been reading the work of Louis Pasteur (1822–1895), a French professor of chemistry and biology. Pasteur believed that microorganisms, or germs in the air, were responsible for food going off and liquids going sour and that rotting and fermenting could occur without air if microorganisms were present.

In 1867, using this knowledge, Lister developed a theory that microorganisms might be causing wound infections. He began to treat wounds by first removing any old clotted blood. Then he soaked the wound in carbolic, before applying a lint which was impregnated with carbolic. On top of this, he placed tinfoil to prevent evaporation, and then packed absorbent wool around the wound. With this combination he aimed to kill any

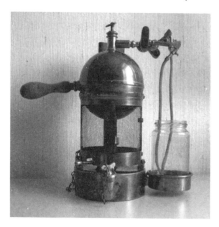

Lister's carbolic acid spray.

germs in the wound and prevent germs from infecting it.

His treatments were successful and he published his results in the *Lancet* on 16th March 1867, showing that in eleven compound fracture cases, where the bone had broken through the skin, none of the patients had died of infection. Lister began to extend his theories to his operating techniques – using carbolic acid to wash his hands before surgery and spraying it around the operating theatre. The death rate fell rapidly, and by the end of the century his technique was being used all over the world.

His ideas about microorganisms weren't widely accepted. Some surgeons were sceptical. John Hughes Bennett, a professor in Edinburgh, said:

'Where are these little beasts? Show them to us, and we shall believe in them. Has anyone seen them yet?'

But Lister remained confident that he was right, and by the 1880s most dissenters were also convinced.

See: *Handwashing*, page 72; *Immunizations*, pages 73–74

Temperature Measurement

Carl Wunderlich (1815–1877)

Measuring the temperature is a fundamental part of medical practice and remains one of the simplest objective measures of illness.

Temperature measurement became possible after the invention of the first thermometer with a scale in 1724 by Gabriel Daniel Fahrenheit (1686–1736), a natural scientist who had also trained as a glass blower. There were three points on Fahrenheit's scale: zero, which was determined by the temperature of a mixture of ice, water and sea salt; 32 degrees, which was the freezing point of water; and 96 degrees, which was the temperature of the human body.

However, it took another century before physicians fully realized the significance of the thermometer in medical practice.

In 1868 Wunderlich, a German physician, published *Das Verhalten der Eigenwarme in Krankheiten* (*The Temperature in Diseases*). In it he presented his readings and analysis from nearly 25,000 patients. This must have taken some time, given that apparently his thermometer was 30cm/1ft long and it took 20 minutes to get a reading! Nonetheless, he recorded temperature variations in over 30 different diseases, concluding that temperature readings could provide information about the disease.

Wunderlich emphasized the importance of getting temperature readings twice a day, to establish a pattern that could be easily interpreted. However, nurses or even relatives could do the readings. These days, mercury thermometers have largely been replaced by infrared measurements of the tympanic membrane in the ear.

Paracetamol

Harmon Northrop Morse (1848–1920)

Paracetamol is a popular painkiller, often used to treat a fever, and also to relieve headaches and minor ailments.

Although Harmon Northrop Morse, a professor of inorganic chemistry in New York's John Hopkins University, discovered paracetamol in 1878, nobody really realized its full significance until about 70 years later.

Two other drugs were used to reduce fever before Paracetamol's significance became known – acetanilide in 1886 and phenacetin in 1887.

In 1893 there was a significant finding when paracetamol crystals were found in the urine of people who had taken phenacetin. This suggested that the body converted phenacetin into paracetamol. Five years later, in 1899, scientists found that acetanilide was also converted to paracetamol.

However, it was not until 1946 that anyone realized that paracetamol was a useful drug. In that year, the American Institute for the Study of Analgesic and Sedative Drugs awarded a grant to the New York City Department of Health to study pain relievers. Chemists Bernard Brodie (1910–1978) and Julius Axelrod (1912–2004), who in 1970 won the Nobel Prize for his contribution to our understanding of neurotransmitters such as adrenaline, were assigned to investigate acetanilide in more detail. They found that it was only when acetanilide was converted to paracetamol in the body that it had its active effect on pain and fever. In a paper, published in 1948, they concluded that paracetamol could be a useful treatment on its own.

Paracetamol is one of the safest drugs for pain relief. But, if the proper dose is exceeded, it can cause liver damage which can be fatal if not treated. Paracetamol is now sold in smaller quantities. with clear warnings about the risks of overdose.

Handwashing

Louis Pasteur (1822–1895)

Surprisingly it wasn't always recognised that diseases could be transmitted by touch.

Ignaz Semmelweis was a doctor working in the obstetrics clinic in Vienna where women went to give birth. In those days childbirth was risky, and of those that survived, many went on to die from an overwhelming infection called puerperal fever shortly afterwards. Giving birth in hospital was more dangerous than being at home: as many as a third of women died from infection in some wards.

Then in 1947, the Professor of Forensic Medicine, while perfoming an autopsy, cut his finger, which became infected, and when the infection spread to his bloodstream, he eventually died. The breakthrough came when Semmelweis realised the professor must have caught the infection from the woman's body and that if this was the case, infections could be transmitted from one woman to the next simply by the touch of the doctor or attending midwife. However, he believed that by handwashing between patients, it should be possible to stop the spread of infection.

So Semmelweis ordered that all the doctors, medical students and midwives should wash their hands with chlorinated water before deliveries, and the death rate immediately plummeted.

Semmelweis' discovery remains one of the most important weapons we have today in the fight against potentially fatal hospital acquired infections, such as MRSA (methicillin-resistant staphylococcus aureus).

Immunizations

Louis Pasteur (1822–1895)

Immunization involves inoculating a small amount of an infectious disease into a healthy person in order to protect them against a disease.

Chemist Louis Pasteur realized that germs were responsible for causing disease and that once these organisms were identified, it would be possible to prevent specific diseases.

Pasteur was born in Dole, France, son of a tanner. He was ambitious, and from the start it was clear that chemistry was his passion. He studied chemistry in Paris, and although one of his tutors called Pasteur 'mediocre', he quickly proved himself in the field. His doctoral thesis on crystallography helped him obtain a position as a professor of chemistry in Strasbourg.

By 1879, Pasteur was working as a professor of chemistry and biology in Lille, France, where he was partly responsible for finding solutions for problems in the manufacture of alcohol locally. His research into beer and wine fermentation led him to believe that there were micro-organisms present in the air, which could be grown and studied.

Once he had begun to identify different types of micro-organisms, and the diseases they caused, Pasteur began to experiment with disease prevention.

In 1879 he injected chickens with cholera bacteria that he had grown several weeks earlier and which had lost some of their strength, to cause illness. The chickens survived. Then Pasteur injected the same birds, and a new batch, with a new and more powerful culture of cholera bacteria. The birds which had previously been injected remained well, whereas the other ones fell ill.

Using the knowledge and experience he gained from dealing with cholera, Pasteur turned his attention to anthrax, an infection in cattle, which also caused a lung disease in woolsorters. In a dramatic public demonstration in 1881, he injected 24 sheep, one goat, and six cows with the anthrax vaccine. A few weeks later he injected anthrax bacteria into the same animals and also into another similar group of animals which had not been previously vaccinated. Three days later, the vaccinated animals had all survived, while the rest were dead.

Pasteur also developed a vaccine against rabies, a terrible disease that is still difficult to treat once it takes hold. The rabies vaccine was first used in humans in 1885.

See: *Smallpox Vaccine*, page 38; *The Eradication of Smallpox*, page 141

Pinard Stethoscope

Adolphe Pinard (1844–1934)

Before modern technology enabled doctors to measure the foetal heartbeat in a pregnant woman, they relied on a simple instrument called a Pinard stethoscope.

The Pinard stethoscope was used widely until the end of the 20th century, when it was replaced by ultrasound monitors. It has a flat earpiece and a wider end for placing on the woman. Traditionally, midwives used the stethoscope to listen to the foetal heartbeat during, and after, every labour contraction.

The first person to describe the sound of the baby's heartbeat before birth was Francois Mayor (1779-1855), a doctor working in Geneva in 1818. However, he did not recognize how this information might be useful for establishing the wellbeing of the unborn child. It was Jean de Kergaredec (1787-1877), a student of Rene Laennec (1781–1826), the inventor of the stethoscope, who published a paper in 1822 explaining the clinical significance of the foetal heart rate.

It took another 60 years before the invention of the Pinard stethoscope, designed specifically for listening to the heart sounds more carefully. The stethoscope took its name from Adolph Pinard, a French obstetrician, who is considered by many to be a pioneer of modern perinatal càre.

Pinard's provision of social care to deprived pregnant women progressed to a recognition of the value of medical care of mother and baby before and after birth.

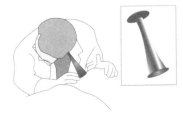

A doctor using a modern Pinard (insert left).

Sphygmomanometer

Samuel Siegfried von Basch (1837–1905)

A sphygmomanometer measures blood pressure and is now an integral part of medical practice. It provides information about a patient's general health, and in particular the state of the heart and blood vessels.

There are two figures in a blood-pressure reading. The top figure, or systolic pressure, is the highest pressure reached as blood is pumped out of the heart. The diastolic, or lower figure, is the resting blood pressure in between beats.

Samuel von Basch, a Czech–Austrian physician, described the first sphygmomanometer in 1881. It was a water-filled bag connected to a manometer (an instrument used for measuring pressure) and it measured the pressure required to stop the arterial pulse in the arm. However it was notoriously inaccurate, and was replaced by a machine made by the Italian physician Scipione Riva-Rocci (1863–1937) in 1896.

Riva-Rocci's device incorporated an armband that could be inflated until it was not possible to feel the pulse below it. As the pressure was released, the pulse returned. The point at which the pulse returned was the systolic pressure and was measured on a mercury manometer attached to the machine.

Riva-Rocci's machine didn't measure diastolic pressure. That came in 1905, when Russian physician Nikolai Korotkoff (1874–1920) suggested using a stethoscope with the sphygmomanometer to listen to blood flow at the same time as measuring the pressure. The systolic pressure is the sound heard when blood flows for the first time through the artery as the pressure is released. The diastolic is when the blood flow sound disappears.

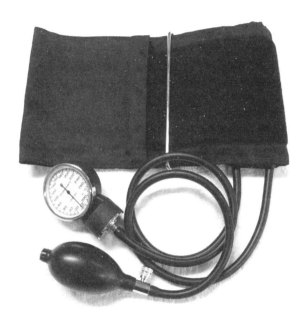

A present-day manual sphygmomanometer.

The American neurosurgeon Harvey Cushing (1869–1939) spotted Riva-Rocci's sphygmomanometer while he was travelling through Italy and recognized its potential. He introduced it to the United States on his return there in 1901, and so it is he who is largely responsible for the instrument's popularity.

The sphygmomanometer has been modified again since then, but, although many doctors now use an electronic version of the instrument, the principle behind it remains unchanged.

Local Anaesthetics

Carl Koller (1857–1944)

Finding a medicine that could make an area of the body numb, such as cocaine, enabled surgeons to carry out treatment without the risk of a general anaesthetic.

The discovery came via the South American Indians who had known for centuries that if they chewed the leaves of the cocoa plant, not only did they feel more alert and less hungry, but it also numbed the mouth and stomach.

However, it was not until 1860 that the German chemist Albert Niemann

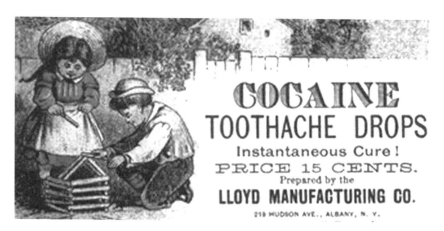

COCAINE TOOTHACHE DROPS
Instantaneous Cure!
PRICE 15 CENTS.
Prepared by the
LLOYD MANUFACTURING CO.
219 HUDSON AVE., ALBANY, N. Y.

Cocaine is now a Class A drug, but it was once a popular painkiller.

(1834–1861) extracted the famous white powder from the dried coca leaves and named it cocaine.

In 1880s Vienna psychoanalyst Sigmund Freud (1856–1939) became interested in cocaine as a treatment for morphine addiction. He suggested the possible use of cocaine as a local anaesthetic to a young German eye surgeon called Carl Koller.

At the time, eye surgery was fraught with difficulty because of the problems of operating on a moving target and of course the pain it caused. However, Koller experimented with cocaine, first on himself, and then on his patients, and found that just a few drops temporarily paralysed the eye movements during surgery and removed pain.

American doctor William Halsted (1852–1922) followed up on Koller's work by experimenting with cocaine injection into nerves to produce local anaesthetic and soon it was also being used to inject under the skin to allow small operations. Unfortunately, Halsted also discovered cocaine's potential for abuse and he spent years trying to overcome his addiction.

In time, cocaine became very popular, and was used for many years in all branches of medicine. Today, it is rarely used, as other safer local anaesthetics with less potential for abuse have emerged. However, it is still produced in vast volumes for recreational use.

See: *General Anaesthetic*, pages 48–49

Contact Lenses

F. E. Muller

It took over 300 years from the original detailed descriptions and drawings of the contact lens by the great artist Leonardo Da Vinci (1452–1519) in 1508 before people began to consider using contact lenses instead of spectacles.

The first person to suggest how to convert the theory into practice was an English astronomer, John Herschel (1792–1871). In 1827 he described a way of grinding a lens out of glass to fit onto the surface of the eye. Sixty years later, in 1887, a German glassblower, F. E. Muller, who made artificial eyes, put Herschel's ideas into practice and produced the first contact lens.

A year later Adolf Eugen Fick (1829–1901), a German physician, described the 'Contactbrille' (a contact spectacle) and fitted them on himself and a group of six patients with good results. At the same time, Paris-based optician, Edouard Kalt, made a similar glass contact lens.

However, these first lenses, being made of glass and quite large, were risky to put in, and were uncomfortable to wear. Glass didn't allow oxygen to pass through to the eye so they weren't good for the health of the tissues, and there was a serious risk of infection. Not surprisingly most people opted to continue wearing their glasses.

Things only began to change after New York optician William Feinbloom (1904–1985) invented hard plastic lenses in 1936. They had a central portion of glass, with plastic around the edge, allowing a bit more oxygen to flow through to the eye, making them less painful to wear, and better for the eyes.

In 1948, Californian optician Kevin Tuohy (1919–1968) began manufacturing contact lenses made completely of plastic. His lenses were smaller than Feinbloom's and later the same year, Oregon optician George Butterfield (1895–1973) improved Tuohy's lens design, adding flatter, peripheral curves to lenses so they were a better fit.

Throughout the 1950s and 1960s, the designs got smaller and thinner and better to wear, but they were largely replaced by modern soft contact lenses finally created in the 1960s by Czechoslovakian chemist, Otto Wichterle (1913–1998) and his assistant Dr Drahoslav Lim (d.2003). Being even thinner and more comfortable than hard contacts, the new softer lenses made the wearing of contact lenses a real possibility for many more people.

Dr Wichterle's work later resulted in the first commercially available soft contact lenses by Bausch & Lomb in 1971.

See: *Spectacles,* pages 21–22; *Ophthalmoscope,* pages 55–56

Electrocardiogram (ECG)

Augustus Désiré Waller (1856–1922)

As is the case with many inventions, the clinical significance of the ECG was not immediately apparent to the inventors. However, it has since proved to be one of the most useful investigative tools to diagnose heart and lung disorders.

The ECG was first described in 1887 by British physiologist Augustus Désiré Waller, who was working at St Mary's Hospital Medical School in London. At the time, there was a lot of interest among his peers in trying to understand more about the electrical activity in the heart.

In 1842, animal experiments by Italian physicist Carlo Matteucci (1811–1868) had shown that an electrical current preceded every heartbeat. Soon everybody, including Waller, was trying to measure these electrical currents.

The electrical current that starts a heartbeat is tiny, and at that time the only way to detect it was by attaching electrodes directly onto the heart. Waller was the first to design a machine that could record this electrical activity using sensors placed on the outside of the body. His equipment included a photographic plate mounted on the chassis of a hand-made toy train and chamois leather-covered zinc electrodes, or sensors attached to the four limbs, with the fifth placed in the mouth. In 1887 he and his laboratory technician, Thomas Goswell, made the first ECG recording.

Apparently, Waller was often accompanied by his bulldog, Jimmy, and in 1909 he gave a lecture about the ECG in front of the Royal Society with Jimmy as the subject, wired to the recording equipment. This prompted irate spectators to write a letter to *The Lancet*,

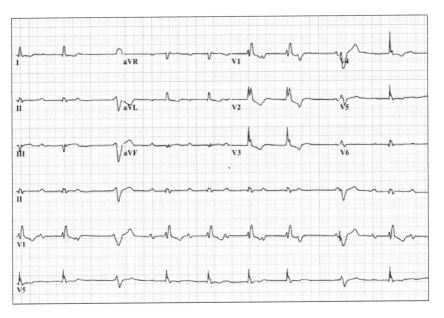

A typical ECG readout.

complaining that the poor dog had undergone '*an ordeal by electricity*'.

The Dutch physiologist Willem Einthoven (1860–1927) further developed Waller's work, distinguishing five different phases (deflections) of electrical current in an electrocardiogram, which he named *P*, *Q*, *R*, *S* and *T*. Willem Einthoven won the Nobel Prize for his work in 1924.

See: *Defibrillator*, pages 93–94

Psychoanalysis

Sigmund Freud (1856–1939)

In the 1880s Freud was a young Viennese neurologist, interested in finding an explanation and treatment for patients suffering from neuroses. His subsequent theory of psychoanalysis has had a lasting influence in the treatment of these patients.

Freud's theories have also played an important role in the history of other disciplines, including art, music, literature, film and philosophy.

Freud was initially influenced by the work of his colleague at the University of Vienna, Dr Josef Breuer (1842–1925), who was interested in the emerging ideas of the unconscious. Breuer used hypnosis as a tool to help patients suffering from hysteria. At the time hysteria was thought to be a neurological disorder, causing a variety of symptoms including paralysis, convulsions, speech abnormalities and blindness. (Some of these cases are now believed to have been caused by epilepsy.)

Famously, Dr Breuer was treating a young woman called Bertha Pappenheim (known better as 'The Case of Anna O'), for symptoms of hysteria. Bertha's symptoms began while she was looking after her dying father. She developed a cough and then other symptoms, including paralysis of the right side of her body, visual disturbances, and lapses of consciousness – symptoms typical of hysteria. Breuer found that he could use hypnosis to allow Bertha to recall her deepest fears and fantasies. He would then discuss these with her when she was not hypnotized and found that the symptoms began to disappear. Bertha called this treatment a talking cure, as if in some way the process of acknowledging her fears led to an improvement in her symptoms.

Freud adapted this technique, encouraging patients to freely associate their thoughts in the presence of the analyst. The idea was that the patient expressed their unconscious thoughts this way. The analyst's role was to interpret these thoughts but without influencing the patient. The patient would lie down on a couch in order to avoid any distraction from their innermost thoughts. Later, Freud developed his ideas to include dream theory and regression to help the patient overcome resistance and uncover hidden unconscious wishes.

He eventually described five fundamental 'pillars' of psychoanalysis: the unconscious, the Oedipus complex, resistance, repression and sexuality. In later years Freud described different stages of development of the human mind: the death instinct, the ego, superego and id.

Freud's ideas gradually spread to France and then to England and America, helped considerably by the Nazis, as many Jewish analysts fled Austria. He was the first person to provide a theoretical basis for mental illness, and his work has had a powerful influence, only challenged by the development of new drug treatments and ECT.

Like many innovators before him, Freud's theories were not universally accepted. Among the dissenters was a Swiss psychiatrist, Carl Gustav Jung (1875–1961), who met Freud in 1907. Jung later founded his own influential movement in analytical psychology.

See: *The Treatment of Epilepsy*, pages 65–66; *Electrocardiogram (ECG)* pages 82–83

Latex Surgical Gloves

William Stewart Halsted (1852–1922)

Surgical gloves help to reduce the risk of infection for patients having surgical procedures.

Gloves used during surgery also protect medical staff from catching something from an infectious patient. However, surgical gloves were not used routinely until the end of the 19th century.

William Stewart Halsted, an American doctor, was convinced of the importance of antisepsis in surgery after a visit by Scottish surgeon Joseph Lister (1827–1912) in 1877. Lister pioneered handwashing and the use of the antiseptic carbolic acid in the operating room after reading Louis Pasteur's (1822–1895) work on micro–organisms and disease.

In 1890, when Halsted was chief surgeon at Johns Hopkins Medical School, the head operating room nurse, Caroline Hampton(born c.1862), complained to him that her hands were sore after using the strong antiseptics for cleaning as he recommended.

So Halsted contacted the Goodyear Rubber Company and commissioned them to make a pair of latex surgical gloves for the soon-to-be Mrs Halsted.

The first gloves reached the elbow. Later his assistant, Joseph Colt Bloodgood (1867–1935) equipped the whole theatre staff with rubber gloves.

For many years, surgical gloves were washed, mended, powdered, sterilized and then reused. It was not until the 1960s that the first disposable natural rubber latex gloves were available for general use.

See: *Handwashing*, page 72; *The Germ Theory of Disease*, pages 68–69

Phototherapy

Niels Finsen (1860–1904)

For thousands of years sunlight has been recognized for its health giving properties. Niels Finsen was the first doctor to carry out scientific experiments on light, showing its beneficial effect, and potential side effects. For his work he was awarded the 1905 Nobel Prize.

Finsen's work was inspired by his own experience of the healing effect of sitting in the sun. He suffered from a hereditary condition called Pick's disease resulting in progressive damage to his internal organs. He died in his early 40s having spent much of his life in a wheelchair.

My disease has played a very great role for my whole development... The disease was responsible for my starting investigations on light: I suffered from anaemia and tiredness ... I began to believe that I might be helped if I received more sun. I therefore spent as much time as possible in its rays. As an enthusiastic medical man I was of course interested to know what benefit the sun really gave.

Physicists already knew that light and heat were part of the electromagnetic spectrum. In 1893 Finsen found that if he exposed smallpox patients to the red light produced by excluding the violet end of the light spectrum, the pustules didn't suppurate or scar. But these got worse when exposed to ultraviolet light. He also found that in some disorders ultraviolet light treatment improved their condition.

By the late 19th century, he was recommending sunbathing as a treatment for tuberculosis. Auguste Rollier (1874–1954), a Swiss doctor who opened several tuberculosis (TB) sanatoriums in the mountains, spread his ideas further.

Röntgen's X-Rays

Karl Wilhelm Röntgen (1845–1923)

The discovery of X-rays provided a window into the body for the first time in history.

Karl Wilhelm Röntgen was a physics professor at Wurzburg University interested in cathode rays. These are carriers of electricity, known as electrons, that travel in a vacuum created inside a glass container from one end to the other when a voltage is applied – otherwise known as a Crookes tube.

Röntgen was working in a darkened laboratory, with the tube wrapped in black cardboard to screen out the light. Switching on the current he noticed that a fluorescent screen nearby glowed brightly. This meant that the Crookes tube was producing some invisible rays capable of passing through the cardboard tube. When he put his hand between the tube and the screen, he saw an image of the bones of his hand on the screen. Experimenting with playing cards, a book, some wood, hard rubber and different kinds of metal, he discovered that the rays would pass through everything except lead.

Röntgen called his discovery X-rays and published his findings in *Über Eine neue Art von Srahlen* (*A New Kind of X-ray*). News of his discovery spread rapidly, and in 1901 he was awarded the Nobel Prize for Physics.

Amid the excitement amongst the medical profession, there was also anxiety that the new discovery could encourage 'peeping toms'. One firm even advertised X-ray proof underwear for protection!

As X-ray technology developed, they began to be used to diagnose broken bones and to locate bullets. Röntgen also discovered that exposure to X-rays could burn the skin, and physicians used this to burn off moles or treat other dermatological conditions.

Facemask

Johannes von Mikulicz-Radecki (1850–1905)

Surgical face masks help to prevent the passage of infection from the surgeon and assistants to the patient.

The modern surgical mask is disposable and made of at least three layers that act as a filter to trap bacteria. The protection lasts for about four hours. The mask covers the nose and is tied around the back of the head.

Modern surgeons wear special operating clothes with hats and boots, together with sterile gowns and gloves in an effort to prevent infection. It wasn't always this way. British surgeon Berkley Moynihan (1865–1936) wrote about what it was like to be a medical student in the 1880s:

The surgeon arrived and threw off his jacket to avoid getting blood or pus on it. He rolled up his shirt-sleeves and, in the corridor to the operation room, took an ancient frock from a cupboard; it bore signs of a chequered past and was utterly stiff with old blood. The cuffs were rolled up to only just above the wrists, and the hands were washed in a sink.

The link between germs and infection came in the late 1870s when German bacteriologist Robert Koch (1843–1910) confirmed and developed the germ theory of disease by culturing and identifying bacteria that caused specific infections.

His results inspired the creation of bacteriology laboratories in hospital clinics and led to the discovery of 'droplet infection' in 1897 by German surgeon Johannes von Mikulicz-Radecki who proved that speaking during operations encouraged infection. He believed this was minimized by wearing face masks.

See: *The Germ Theory of Disease,* pages 68–69

Aspirin

Felix Hoffmann (1868–1946)

Aspirin is known both as a painkiller and for its ability to reduce a fever and limit inflammation. At low doses it also reduces the risk of heart attacks and strokes.

In 1853 French chemist Charles Friedric Gerhardt (1816–1856) was the first person to identify the chemical structure of the active ingredient in Meadowsweet, a natural source of aspirin and well-known folk medicine used to relieve pain. However, the active ingredient, salicylic acid, irritated the stomach lining, causing symptoms of indigestion.

In 1897 Felix Hoffmann of the Bayer drug company found that by converting salicylic acid to acetylsalicylic acid, it became less problematic for the stomach and still worked as a medicine. Two years later the German drug company Bayer began marketing its new product as 'Aspirin'.

It was only during the 1970s that British scientist John Vane (1927–2004) discovered that aspirin also blocks an enzyme needed by the body to produce natural hormones, called prostaglandins, which are involved in many body processes, including pain and tissue injury. In 1982 Professor Vane won the Nobel Prize for Medicine.

Since then many studies have shown that a small dose of aspirin taken daily helps prevent the recurrence of strokes and heart attacks in people already suffering from cardiovascular disease, or who have had a stroke. Scientists believe that this is due to aspirin's effect on prostaglandins by making the platelets less sticky. Platelets are cells in the blood responsible for forming clots. With a daily aspirin, spontaneous clot formation in small blood vessels is less likely, ensuring the passage of oxygen-rich blood to the heart, brain and other body tissues.

Please note: *Always take medical advice before taking a daily dose of aspirin.*

Blood Groups

Karl Landsteiner (1868–1943)

In 1897 Landsteiner found that every person has blood from groups A, B or O. The fourth main blood group, AB, was revealed a year later.

———————

Karl Landsteiner's categorization of blood groups helped make blood transfusions safer.

Prior to this, blood transfusion was a dangerous, often fatal treatment, used as a last resort in patients who had haemorrhaged, particularly after childbirth. Landsteiner studied medicine in Vienna, graduating in 1891, before going on to study chemistry and immunity in more depth.

Working in the University of Vienna as an assistant, Landsteiner found that every person had a blood group that depended on the presence or absence of certain chemical structures – known as antigens on the surface of the red cells – and the natural antibodies in the bloodstream. He

Blood group	Antigen on red blood cells	Antibody in plasma	Can give blood to	Can accept blood from
A	A	anti-B	A and AB	A and O
B	B	anti-A	B and AB	B and O
AB	A and B	neither	AB	all groups
O	neither	anti-A and anti-B	all groups	O

realized that blood transfusion would only be safe if the blood groups of the donated blood and the patient were compatible.

Landsteiner won the Nobel Prize for physiology and medicine in 1930 for his work on blood groups. It's typical of Landsteiner's commitment to his work that he was still working in the laboratory at the age of 75, when he had a heart attack, from which he died two days later.

DONOR

RECIPIENT	O	A	B	AB
AB	♥	♥	♥	♥
B	♥		♥	
A	♥	♥		
O	♥			

This diagram demonstrates the compatibility, or otherwise, of different blood groups from the original donor to the recipient.

Defibrillator

Jean-Louis Prévost (1838–1927)
Frédéric Batelli (1867–1941)

Although the defibrillators used today originated in the 20th century, the use of electric shock in reviving patients dates back centuries.

The electric charge delivered by a defibrillator machine can convert a heart that's not beating into a normal healthy rhythm and prevent sudden death.

In 1788 Charles Kite (1769–1811), member of the Royal Humane Society of London, described the case of a small child who had fallen out of a window. A local doctor, with the aid of an electric shock, revived her. Kite described it as follows:

Twenty minutes had at least elapsed before he could apply the shock, which he gave to various parts of the body without any apparent success; but at length, on transmitting a few shocks through the thorax, he perceived a small pulsation; soon after the child began to breathe, though with great difficulty. In about 10 minutes she vomited. A kind of stupor remained for some days; but the child was restored to perfect health and spirits in about a week.

Modern day-defibrillator machines didn't emerge until the 20th century. Their development was based on work done by two Swiss professors, Jean-Louis Prévost and Frédéric Batelli. In 1899 these two men found that they could bring on a life- threatening abnormal heart rhythm (ventricular fibrillation) in dogs with a small electric shock, and that larger charges would restore the normal rhythm, or defibrillate the heart.

Prévost and Batelli's defibrillator didn't become popular until nearly 50 years later when an American surgeon – Claude Beck – used a similar machine to resuscitate a 14-year-old boy during open heart surgery using elecrodes that delivered 300 volts directly into the heart.

Clearly, defibrillating directly onto the heart during open heart surgery is a technique with limited use. So this was not used much until the invention of a defibrillator that could be used on the outside of the the body a year later in Russia.

By the 1960s, the external defibrillator design had improved, and a portable version that could be used in ambulances now became available.

The most up-to-date versions of defibrillators are fully automated. The rhythm can be analysed by the machine via the electrodes placed on the patient's chest. The machine will also decide whether an electrical shock will help restore normal heart rhythm, so it is possible for bystanders to use the machines without any previous clinical knowledge. Portable, fully automated defibrillators are now found in railway stations, aeroplanes and even in some supermarkets.

See: *Electrocardiogram (ECG), pages 82–83*

Corneal Grafting

Eduard Zirm (1863–1944)

*Scarring or disease in the clear part of the eye
in front of the iris and pupil known as the cornea
is a common cause of permanent blindness.
Transplanting a healthy cornea from an organ
donor can restore normal vision.*

Austrian Ophthalmologist Eduard Zirm pioneered corneal transplants.

Alois Glogar, a labourer who had scarred his eyes from accidental burns, came to see Zirm in Olomouc in Austria. There was little the surgeon could do at that time to help. However, soon after this Zirm saw an 11-year-old boy, Karl Brauer (born c.1894), who had been in an accident that resulted in some pieces of metal penetrating his eye. Unfortunately it was not possible to save Brauer's eye, but the cornea was not damaged. Realizing the potential for the healthy cornea, Zirm transplanted the tissue into Glogar's eyes. Although one eye did not do well, the other recovered, enabling Glogar to return to work.

Since Zirm's breakthrough, advances in microscopes have allowed surgeons to operate more easily on the eye. Together with improved sutures and specialist drugs to combat graft rejection, the success rates of corneal transplants are now very encouraging.

The procedure involves removing a circular disc of the damaged cornea, and replacing it with a disc the same size of the donated healthy cornea, held in place with tiny stitches. After a few days with an eye patch, and steroid drops, in most cases the vision will gradually return to normal.

Corneal tissue has the advantage over most other transplantable organs in that it can be removed up to 24 hours after death, and there is no upper age limit for donors, so there are more potential donors than for other organs. An international network of 'eye banks', or organizations coordinates the distribution of donated corneas to eye surgeons.

Anyone who wishes to donate his or her corneas is required to complete an organ donor registration form.

Corneal grafting.

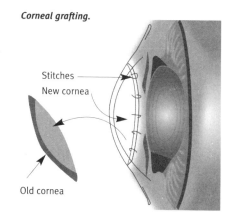

Stitches

New cornea

Old cornea

Discovery of Alzheimer's Disease

Alois Alzheimer (1864–1915)

A gradual decline in mental capacity is recognized as part of the normal ageing process. However, in some cases it is more dramatic, and leads to the crumbling of any recognizable personality as it progresses to dementia. This is called Alzheimer's Disease.

In the early 20th century, the pathological process responsible for the condition was identified in the brain tissue.

Alois Alzheimer was a German psychiatrist and neuropathologist. His original thesis was on the wax-producing glands of the ear, but fortunately for humankind, he moved on to weightier subjects!

After he qualified as a doctor he spent five months working in Frankfurt Asylum. While he was there, he observed a 51-year-old woman, Auguste Deter, who was experiencing strange symptoms, including short-term memory loss, hallucinations, disorientation and difficulty in understanding questions. When she died

five years later in 1906, Alzheimer had both the patient records and brain sent to Munich, Germany, where he was working. Using newly developed techniques to look at pathological samples under the microscope, he was able to identify specific abnormalities in Mrs Deter's brain, which we now know are typical of Alzheimer's.

First Alzheimer found that the brain tissue was thinner than normal. He also found structures called senile plaques, which are typically found in elderly patients. Thirdly, he described twisted bands of fibres – neurofibillary tangles – which had not previously been seen in the brain. It was this last abnormality which defined the disease.

Most people who are diagnosed with

Brain Cross-Sections

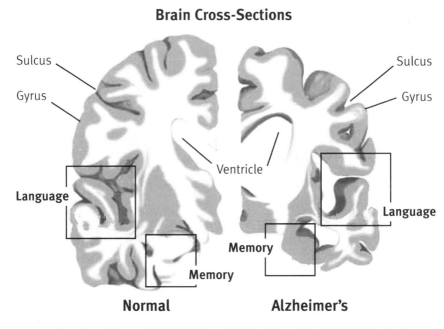

A comparison of part of a normal, healthy brain on the left with one affected by Alzheimer's Disease on the right.

Alzheimer's disease develop it after the age of 65 years. However, there is a rare inherited form, which affects less than 1 in 10 people with the disease and develops in adults before age 65. In such cases, there is a 50 per cent chance of developing the disease in all of the children of the affected parent.

Although the diagnosis of Alzheimer's Disease can still only be made by post-mortem examination of the brain to confirm the presence of these abnormal patterns, doctors can now make an accurate diagnosis most of the time by careful questioning and examination, incorporating detailed memory and psychological tests, while the patient is still alive. Early diagnosis is now more important than ever since the advent of new medications, which slow the progression of this very destructive disease.

Contraceptive Coils

Richard Richter

*This reliable form of contraception is now
used by 100 million women worldwide.*

———

The first known Intrauterine device
(IUD) was designed by Dr R. Richter,
a German gynaecologist, in 1909, and
consisted of two strands of silkworm gut
wound together and shaped into a ring.

The free ends were capped with
celluloid to prevent them from injuring
the lining of the uterus and poked
through the cervix so that the device
could be removed easily.

Richter's invention did not have any
impact on the practice of birth control.
It wasn't until Karl P. Ernst Gräfenberg
(1881–1957), a German gynaecologist,
invented the Ring IUD that things
began to change. Speaking in 1929 in
London, where he presented his
invention, he said:

*'A satisfactory contraceptive method
is most important in dealing with
psychosexual disturbances in
women. By removing fear and the
necessity for objectionable
preparations, many physical and
mental inhibitions are removed.'*

Gräfenberg reported a pregnancy rate
of just 8 per cent in 1,100 women using
his ring, and the following year when he
modified the design to incorporate silver
wire wrapped around the coil, he
reported a 1.6 per cent pregnancy rate in
600 women. What Dr Gräfenberg didn't
know is that the silver wire was
contaminated with 26 per cent copper.
Copper increased the effectiveness of
the IUD, but that wasn't recognized for
another 40 years.

Thirty years later, Gräfenberg was
the first person to describe the vaginal
erogenous zone, which was named the
'G-spot' after him!

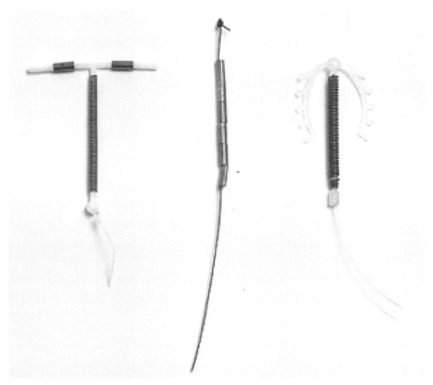

A selection of contraceptive coils.

Later developments in IUD technology have led to refinements in the design. Plastic IUDs were introduced in the 1950s, copper was added in the 1960s and progesterone-releasing coils appeared in 1996.

See: *Condoms*, pages 17–18

The Band-Aid

Earle Dickson (1892–1961)

It is virtually impossible to imagine treating a blister or small cut these days without being able to reach for an adhesive plaster. They are part of our everyday lives.

When Earle Dickson got married in 1917, his wife Josephine had a succession of minor cuts while preparing food and all he could do was provide a big clumsy bandage.

At the time, he was working as a cotton buyer for the family firm Johnson & Johnson, set up by the Johnson brothers Robert, James and Edward in 1885 to produce surgical dressings.

Dickson worked away on producing a better dressing to help his wife by folding sterile gauze in the centre of a strip of surgical tape, and then covering the strip with a piece of crinoline to prevent the tape from sticking to itself, before rolling it up again. She could subsequently cut off what she needed next time there was an injury.

Dickson persuaded his company to make his design commercially and they called it Band-Aid.

Although at first it did not sell very well, things picked up after Johnson & Johnson distributed free Band-Aids to Boy Scouts troupes across the United States. By 1924 there was a range of sizes and shapes available. Shortly afterwards, Elastoplast appeared in the UK, and the rest is history.

The Operating Microscope

Carl Olof Nylén (1892–1978)

Visualizing delicate structures within the body has become much easier since the invention of the operating microscope. It has also made it possible to carry out more complex reconstructive surgery and neurosurgery.

Before the invention of the operating microscopes, surgeons relied on the strength of their own vision to operate on tiny structures. This limited what they could do, and often led to them accidentally damaging delicate organs.

In 1921, Nylén, an Ear, Nose and Throat surgeon, invented a simple microscope to use in his operating theatre at the Ear Nose and Throat clinic in Stockholm where he worked. It had one eyepiece and was rapidly replaced by a binocular microscope (with two eyepieces) invented by his boss, Gunnar Holmgren (1875–1954).

However, Holmgren's microscope was a poor quality instrument with an inadequate light source, so was not widely used until a new model appeared in 1951 developed by physicist Hans Littman and the Zeiss Company founded by Carl Zeiss, a German optician.

The quality was so much better that ophthalmologists, vascular, plastic and neurosurgeons began using it regularly. By looking through the microscope, the surgeon was now able to view more detail in the operating site, enabling more accuracy during the procedure. Very quickly operating using microscopes became standard practice.

Insulin

Sir Frederick Banting (1891–1941)

The discovery of insulin has saved the lives of many millions of diabetics with insulin dependent (or type 1) diabetes and has been one of the 20th century's most significant medical breakthroughs.

During digestion the body normally changes sugars and other nutrients into a form of sugar called glucose. The blood carries glucose to cells in the body and insulin helps change it into energy for cells to use. We rely for survival on this ability to change food into energy.

Type 1 diabetics cannot digest sugar due to a lack of insulin, which is normally produced in the pancreas. As a result, the blood sugar level is high, and people with this condition feel tired and thirsty, lose weight and pass large quantities of sugary urine. Diabetes is rapidly fatal unless treated with insulin.

Although German researchers had already discovered, back in 1889, that the pancreas contained something that stopped diabetes from developing, attempts to isolate this substance and use it for treatment were unsuccessful.

It was only made possible 30 years later, when John Mcleod, professor of physiology in Toronto, gave Frederick Banting, a surgeon at the hospital, and a medical student called Charles Best, the run of his laboratory while he went fishing in Scotland for the summer. Working with dogs in the laboratory, the men incorporated the work of a biochemist called James Bertram Collip who began refining a pure extract of the pancreas containing the anti-diabetic agent later known as insulin.

Leonard Thompson, a 14-year-old diabetic, was the first human to receive the pure extract. Thompson had been diabetic for three years and at the time he was near death, weighing just 65 pounds. After receiving Collip's extract, Thompson's symptoms began to disappear and his blood sugar returned to normal. The results were unequivocal; this extract of pancreas had a significant anti-diabetic effect on humans.

The new extract was called insulin and began to be produced in industrial quantities by Eli Lilly in Indianapolis.

In recognition of their achievement, the 1923 Nobel Prize in Physiology and Medicine was awarded to Banting and Macleod who shared the money with Best and Collip.

EEG

Hans Berger (1873–1941)

The brain generates electrical activity which can be recorded on a graph.

Hans Berger had originally wanted to be an astronomer. While in the army, he narrowly escaped serious injury when his horse slipped down a steep slope. His sister, although miles away, felt aware that her brother was in danger, and sent him a telegram. Berger was so amazed by this, that he switched to psychology and later to medicine. He specialised in the study of brain function, becoming a neuropsychologist at a time when most things were learnt about the body from dissecting it.

He had read about the work by Richard Caton (1842–1926), a Liverpool surgeon who was studying brain activity in animals, and it convinced him that the human brain also produced electrical impulses. He went on to become the first person to prove their existence using his invention, which he called an 'elektroenkephalogramm', or EEG, that recorded brain waves on a graph.

In his research Berger made 73 EEG recordings from his son Klaus, aged 15. He described a particular type of wave, which he called the 'Berger' waves, (now renamed 'Alpha' waves), that were present when the eyes were closed. When the eyes were open the waves changed and these are known as 'long' or 'beta' waves.

Berger's publication of *On the Electroencephalogram of Man* in 1929 and his invention of the EEG was the start of a change in the understanding of brain diseases, such as epilepsy, and has helped to provide a better understanding of how the brain works, as well as how to recognize abnormalities in brain function.

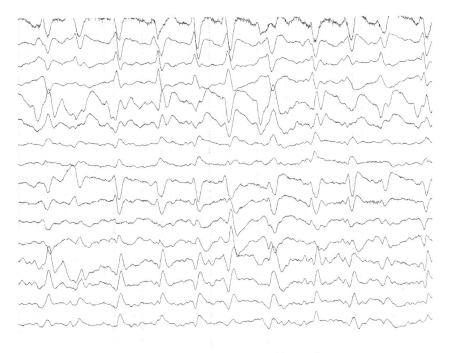

Electrical brain activity, as captured in an EEG.

The National Blood Transfusion Service

A network of centres providing quick access to safe blood for transfusing into patients with severe blood loss has been a lifesaver for millions of people worldwide.

Although doctors had experimented with blood transfusion before the 20th century, particularly in their efforts to save women who had haemorrhaged in childbirth, their attempts were usually unsuccessful. Few people survived a transfusion, but nobody was sure why it was so dangerous.

In 1897, Karl Landsteiner (1868–1943) was the first to discover that there are different blood groups, A, B and O. A fourth blood group, AB, was discovered a year later. Later three more blood groups were found, M, N and P, as well as the Rhesus blood groups. Only certain combinations are safe to mix together. Understanding this meant that it was possible to learn how to transfuse like for like blood from one person to another.

Even after Landsteiner's discovery, it took some years before blood transfusion became established practice, partly because the techniques for collecting blood and stopping it from clotting had not been fully established.

During the First World War (1914–1918), doctors discovered that it was possible to prevent blood from clotting after it was removed from the body by mixing it with sodium citrate. They also discovered they could keep blood supplies for longer if they were refrigerated. Many wounded soldiers benefited from this knowledge.

The first voluntary blood service began in 1921 when the British Red Cross members all gave blood at Kings College Hospital, London, and then in 1926, they set up the first blood transfusion service.

Electrosurgery

William T. Bovie (1882–1958)

Using an instrument delivering high-frequency electric current to create heat provided a new method for controlling bleeding during surgery, and for cutting tissue without significant blood loss.

This technique expanded the possibilities for surgery, allowing surgeons to undertake procedures that were previously considered too dangerous due to the risks of bleeding.

Heat has been used to seal blood vessels since 3,000 BC. However, generating heat through electricity only began in the late 19th century, when it was discovered that high-frequency current created heat without damaging or stimulating the tissues.

Bovie, a physicist working at Harvard University, developed a device that the famous neurosurgeon Harvey Cushing (1869–1939) used to remove a tumour. The patient had a tumour growing on his head that Cushing had unsuccessfully tried to remove already, having had to abandon

surgery due to excessive bleeding.

After reoperating using Bovie's electrosurgical instrument, Cushing wrote:

...with Dr Bovie's help I proceeded to take off most satisfactorily the remaining portion of tumor with practically none of the bleeding which was occasioned in the preceding operation.

Early electrosurgical units became popular in operating rooms all over the world and were often referred to as 'the bovie' by the operating surgeon.

Despite its success, Bovie received nothing: he sold his patent to the Liebel-Flarsheim company of Cincinnati for $1.19 and was not even granted tenure at Harvard.

Iron Lung

Louis Agassiz Shaw (1886–1940)
Philip Drinker (1894–1972)

Before the introduction of the polio vaccine in the 1950s, polio was a common disease. In the early stages of the disease it paralysed the breathing muscles and many patients died.

———

The invention of the artificial breathing machine, nicknamed 'the iron lung', allowed doctors to keep patients breathing for long enough for recovery to take place. Those that survived recovered most or all of their earlier strength.

This is how one patient described the experience of having polio:

'When I first contracted polio, except for my arms, hands, and neck muscles, I seemed to have paralysis all over my body. My taste buds were affected; my eyes refused to focus correctly; my mind wandered; and lung muscles were also stricken. At the end of six weeks, I lifted my head off the pillow and was able to sneeze slightly. Three weeks [later] I managed to turn myself on my side. By this time I was able to carry on a conversation without running out of breath. In December, my feet returned for the most part to a normal condition.' (Mrs. V.A. Pahl, 1940s).

In 1640, John Mayo, a British lawyer and chemist who then became a doctor, was the first to demonstrate the mechanics of breathing. He showed that air was sucked into the lungs when the walls of the chest expanded and the diaphragm became flat. He built a model using bellows with a bladder inside to illustrate his theory. By expanding the bellows, air was drawn into the bladder, and compressing the bellows forced the air out of the bladder.

Understanding this principle of 'external negative pressure ventilation' allowed Philip Drinker and Louis Agassiz Shaw to build a modern version in 1927 that became the first iron lung. Using an electric motor and two vacuum cleaners, they built a machine capable of keeping a patient's breathing going until they could breathe on their own again, which usually took one or two weeks.

The patient had to lie flat on their back with only their head visible. There was a rubber collar forming a comfortable, yet tight seal around their neck. Their machine was a success, and in 1927, the first iron lung was installed at Bellevue hospital in New York.

President Franklin Delano Roosevelt (1882–1945), who had himself had polio, was an ardent supporter of medical research on the prevention and treatment of polio.

In 1938, he established the National Foundation for Infantile Paralysis to encourage the search for a polio vaccine. Supported by funding from the Foundation, iron lungs were widely distributed throughout the United States from 1939.

Discovery of Penicillin

Alexander Fleming (1881–1955)

Before the discovery of penicillin, even a scratch could be fatal if it became infected.

Alexander Fleming studied medicine at St Mary's Hospital in London, qualifying with the top marks in his year. After serving in the Medical Corps in the First World War (1914–1918), he returned to the medical school, eventually becoming professor, while also undertaking medical research.

It was while Fleming was working in the research laboratories at St Mary's hospital in 1928 that he first discovered penicillin. At the time, he was studying a germ called staphylococcus, responsible for boils, abscesses and carbuncles. On his return from holiday, he found that some mould had contaminated and destroyed the staphylococcus culture.

After a few more experiments, Fleming found that this happened even when he diluted the mould 800 times. And although the mould attacked the bacteria, it did not have the same effect on all germs and, crucially, had no toxic effect on healthy tissues. Fleming was unable to separate the active substance from the mould but he did name it penicillin.

More than 10 years elapsed before the next development in the story. In Oxford England, the Australian pathologist Howard Florey (1898–1968) set up a team of scientists, including Ernst Chain (1906–1979), a refugee from Nazi Germany, to study substances capable of blocking the effect of microorganisms such as staphylococcus. The team discovered a technique for isolating penicillin. Then they purified it until they had collected enough to test it first in mice, and then in humans.

When drug companies started mass production, many thousands of servicemen benefited from treatment of war wounds with penicillin at the end of the Second World War (1939–1945).

In recognition of their groundbreaking contribution to medical science, Chain, Florey and Fleming were awarded the 1945 Nobel Prize in Medicine.

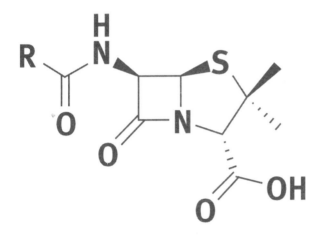

The chemical structure of the core of penicillin.

Wheelchair

Herbert B. Everest
Harry C. Jennings

Although chairs had been adapted with wheels before, Everest's and Jennings's invention was the first folding, self-propelled wheelchair.

The first known wheelchair was invented over 400 years ago for Phillip II of Spain (1527–1598). A 1595 drawing of the king shows him in a chair with wheels, arm-rests and foot-rests. The arms of the chair are hinged and there are ratchets to adjust the angle of the back and legs. However, this chair wasn't self-propelled.

In 1665, a paralysed German watchmaker invented a wheelchair with three wheels and a mechanism for moving the chair forward by hand cranks attached to the front wheel.

In 1869, the first patent was granted in the United States for a wheelchair. This chair had a fixed frame, with adjustable parts, a wicker seat and large rear wheels that you could propel forward.

However, it was not until the 20th century that the prototype of the modern wheelchair was invented.

Herbert Everest and Harry Jennings were good friends, and when Everest was paralysed in a mining accident, Jennings, who was a mechanical engineer, set about designing a chair that Everest could move himself, and that could be folded when not in use. The design incorporated a light outer wheel with a slightly smaller circumference, allowing the person in the chair to control the wheelchair without getting their hands dirty. It also used wire-spoked wheels, which had replaced wooden ones in 1900.

The chair was so successful that they

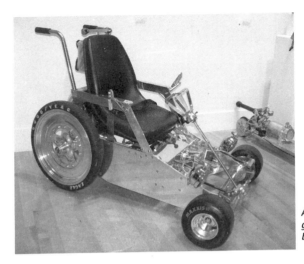

A present-day, avant-garde model, powered by rockets!

began to make more for other people initially by hand in their own garage, making them quite an expensive option. However, the Second World War (1939–1945) provided an influx of paralysed young men looking for suitable wheelchairs. Everest and Jennings had by now formed a company, and this monopolized the market for many years.

Thrombolysis

William Smith Tillett (1892–1974)

Until quite recently there was no treatment for a heart attack, and it was often fatal. However, with the advent of thrombolysis, also known as 'clot busting' drugs, mortality rates fell rapidly.

In 1933 William Tillett, Associate Professor of Medicine and Director of the Biological Division at Johns Hopkins University, discovered almost by accident that streptococci bacteria produced a substance called streptokinase that would break down and clear a blood clot in an artery.

Tillett's discovery inspired research spanning the next 50 years to find the best therapeutic applications for this finding. Gradually, it became clear that an intravenous infusion of streptokinase given to a patient soon after a heart attack might increase the chances of survival.

However, there were some conflicting study findings so although streptokinase was being used to treat heart attacks, it was not widespread. Finally in 1986, the evidence finally arrived. It came from a huge study involving more than 11,000 patients in 176 different coronary care units, and was published in *The Lancet*.

The GISSI study (*Gruppo Italiano per la Sperimentazione della Streptochinasi nell'Infarto Miocardico*) confirmed that treatment with streptokinase significantly reduced mortality after a heart attack and that the sooner treatment was administered, the better the outcome.

Further research has shown that another drug called 'tissue plasminogen activator (t-PA)' is better than streptokinase because patients who receive it live longer. Since the late 1990s, t-PA has been the drug of choice but because it is a more expensive option, streptokinase continues to be the most readily available treatment worldwide.

Pulse Oximeter

Karl Matthes (1931–1998)

Doctors have always relied on looking at the colour of a patient's skin to assess their health. Poor oxygen levels make the lips and fingernails go blue, indicating a serious problem. The Pulse Oximeter is a simple device, a bit like a clothes peg that is clipped onto a finger and measures the amount of oxygen in the blood.

Before the invention of the pulse oximeter, making an accurate assessment of the patient's blood oxygen level required an arterial blood sample, which is an uncomfortable and fiddly investigation. The pulse oximeter has changed all that – and is now regarded as an essential piece of equipment in assessing critically ill patients.

The Oximeter's development began with a German physicist and chemist – Ernest Felix Hoppe Seyler (1825–1895) in the 1860s. He discovered that the pigment in red blood cells, known as haemoglobin, combines with oxygen to form oxyhaemoglobin and that this results in a change in its colour from dark to bright red. Essentially, the modern pulse oximeter measures the colour of the blood and calculates the amount of oxygen in the blood.

The oximeter would not have been developed if it hadn't also been for the spectroscope, invented by the German chemist Robert W. E. Bunsen (1811–1899) and his physicist colleague Gustaf R. Kirchoff (1824–1887) in Heidelberg in 1859. The spectroscope disperses light into a spectrum, allowing it to be analysed.

Although the German physician Karl von Vierordt (1818–1884) used the spectroscope to demonstrate oxygen consumption in his hand in 1876, his results were largely ignored and it was not until the Second World War (1939–1945) that developments continued, spurred on by the need to monitor blood oxygen levels in fighter pilots who tended to black out at high altitudes.

In 1935, Karl Matthes, a Viennese physiologist, introduced the first oximeter. It was clipped onto the earlobe, and was capable of continuously monitoring blood oxygen saturation. However, the device did not take account of the pulsatile nature of blood in arteries, and was cumbersome.

Modified versions of Matthes's original device culminated in the Japanese inventor Takuo Aoyagi's first commercial pulse oximeter in 1974. His device, also clipped to the ear lobe, works on the same principle as the oximeters available today. It derives oxygen content from analysing multiple wavelengths of light, and is independent of the thickness of the ear, the colour of the skin, and the intensity of the light.

Dialysis

Willem Kolff (b. 1911)

Inventor Willem Kolff was inspired to make a machine that could do the work of the kidneys after caring for a young man dying slowly of kidney failure.

Millions of people have benefited from the dialysis machine and are alive today because of it.

Kolff was a young doctor working in The Netherlands when the Second World War (1939–1945) began. He was sent to work in a remote Dutch hospital after the Nazis invaded, where all materials were in short supply and local manufacturers were forbidden to do business with anyone but the occupying army.

Nonetheless, he was resourceful enough to find the materials he needed, making his first dialysis machine out of cellophane tubing wrapped around a cylinder, which would rest in a bath of cleaning fluid. Essentially the patient's blood was drawn into the tubing, into the bath, cleaned and then passed back into the patient's body.

In 1943, Kolff's invention, although crude, was completed. The first patients he treated with no success. But then in 1945 his first patient, a comatose 67-year-old woman, regained consciousness after dialysis and went on to live for another seven years.

The dialysis treatment that Kolff pioneered has saved the lives of hundreds of thousands of men, women and children all over the world.

Sunscreen

Franz Greiter

Sunscreen protects the skin from the harmful effects of ultraviolet radiation from the sun.

Getting a suntan has been popular since the time of the Ancient Greeks, who even had a sun God called Helios. At other times in history, dark skin has been associated with the lower social classes. In Jane Austin's *Pride and Prejudice* (published in 1813), the main protaganist Elizabeth Bennett's naturally olive skin was considered too dark and less attractive as a result.

In the 20th century, with the increase in foreign travel, dark-tanned skin became more popular, and with it came an increase in skin cancers.

The sun emits light, heat (infrared) and ultraviolet A (UVA), B (UVB) and C (UVC) rays. UVA causes skin damage, leading to premature ageing, and UVB causes skin cancer. UVC rays are dispersed into the atmosphere before they reach the earth.

Levels of ultraviolet radiation are much higher at altitude – 4 per cent more per 30m/1000ft, a fact Greiter learned from experience in 1938 when he sustained severe sunburn while climbing Piz Buin, a mountain in the Swiss–Austrian border nearly 11,000 feet high. The ultraviolet radiation would therefore have been 44 per cent more than at ground level. As a keen chemistry student, Greiter set to work on developing a product to protect the skin. His cream, initially called Gletcher Crème (Glacier Cream), later became known as PIZ BUIN®. The original version was only providing low protection but it was the first to provide any at all.

Later, an airman called Benjamin Green developed Red Vet Pet (for red veterinary petrolatum), during the Second World War (1939–1945) when soldiers serving in the Pacific were suffering from sun exposure. The product was sticky, red and not that effective. It worked on the principle of providing a thick layer to block out the sun's rays.

Randomized–Controlled Trial

Austin Bradford Hill (1897–1991)

The randomized–controlled trial is now the cornerstone of medical research. People enrolled into the study are randomly allocated to receive one of several possible treatments. The idea is that provided there are enough people in each group, they should each be a representative sample of the larger population. If that's the case, then the study findings can be applied more generally.

Before the introduction of the randomized–controlled trial, as each patient was recruited to a trial, the researcher would alternate between assigning him or her to one or the other of two (usually no more) treatments. The researcher knew what treatment the last patient had received, and therefore also what the next one would get. This practice meant that researchers might influence whether or when to enter patients into a trial, which is known as selection bias.

Hill was a statistician at the Medical Research Council. He is also famous for his pioneering work with Richard Doll (1912–2005) in linking smoking and lung cancer. His landmark study 'Streptomycin Treatment of Pulmonary Tuberculosis' published in the *British Medical Journal* on 30 October 1948 was the first randomized–controlled trial.

In the trial patients received streptomycin with bed rest, or just bed rest. As a patient was enrolled into the study a sealed envelope was opened with a card marked S for streptomycin or C for control which was be bed rest only. The cards were randomly allocated and there were an equal number of each S and C cards. This design meant it was possible to avoid patient selection bias.

Randomised–controlled trials are widely accepted as good research practice.

Mammography

Raul Leborgne

A mammogram is an X-ray of the breast used to detect breast cancer in women before the cancer causes symptoms. Breast cancer affects more than one in ten women at some stage in their lives.

As early as 1913, a German surgeon called Albert Salman took X-rays of mastectomy specimens, and noticed that it was possible to distinguish different types of breast cancer according to their appearance on the X-ray. This idea was developed further in 1930 when Stafford Warren, a New York based radiologist reported on X-ray images taken before surgery in women with breast cancer, looking for patterns.

Throughout the 1930s a number of doctors made studies of the possible uses of X-rays for examining the breasts, but in 1949, Uruguayan Raul Leborgne was the first to emphasize the need for breast compression during the procedure to identify small areas of calcification which showed up as speckles on the mammogram, often indicating the presence of a cancerous tumour.

In the mid-1950s, Jacob Gershon-Cohen (1899–1971), a radiologist based in Philadelphia, screened healthy women for breast cancer, popularizing the technique. Some remained critical, however, because of the exposure to potentially harmful X-rays that mammograms involved. However, Houston radiologist Robert Egan was instrumental in improving the technical quality of mammograms in the 1950s, which were therefore easier to interpret and safer to use.

In 1963 the first randomized–controlled trial of screening by mammography was carried out in New York showing that mammography reduced the death rate from breast cancer by nearly a third in the five years after the test.

Amniocentesis

Douglas Charles Aitchison Bevis (1919–1994)

Before 1950 there was no screening during pregnancy. With the advent of amniocentesis it became possible to diagnose some diseases before birth.

Although Douglas Bevis's research was published by *The Lancet* in 1950, its significance went unrecognized for at least 10 years.

Bevis was a junior doctor at St Mary's Hospital in London when he carried out his ground-breaking research. The room where he lived in the hospital resembled a research laboratory. It was there that he analysed the content of amniotic fluid samples removed by amniocentesis from pregnant women to determine the possibility of the foetus having a potentially fatal blood disorder known as Haemolytic Disease of the Newborn. This serious condition occurs because of Rhesus blood group incompatibility between mother and baby.

At first during amniocentesis, the doctor had nothing to guide the needle into the uterus, and risked damaging the placenta or growing foetus. After the introduction of obstetric ultrasound, the doctor could see an image of the needle inside the uterus, therefore reducing the risks.

Developments in prenatal diagnosis now allow doctors to use amniocentesis to determine the sex of the baby and diagnose many disorders, including Downs' syndrome.

While the use of amniocentesis to obtain samples of amniotic fluid was available at least 30 years before Bevis published his work, his research into its use in prenatal diagnosis is considered to be a landmark in this field of medicine.

Pacemaker

John A. Hopps (1919–1998)

A pacemaker is a battery-operated device that stimulates the heart to beat regularly by sending electrical impulses via electrodes placed next to the heart wall. The aim is to maintain an adequate heart rate, either because the heart's own pacemaker is too slow, or there is a block in the heart's normal electrical conduction system.

The first mechanical pacemaker was invented in 1926 when Mark Lidwell, an Australian anaesthetist, used it to resuscitate a newborn infant. However he did not patent his idea so does not get the historical credit.

In 1932 American cardiologist Albert Hyman (1893–1972) first successfully used a similar device and coined the term 'artificial pacemaker'. But there was public opposition to the idea. People thought that the machine would be used to wake up the dead. So he didn't pursue his invention in humans, preferring to stick to animal research.

Meanwhile, Canadian electrical engineer Dr John A. Hopps was researching hypothermia and discovered that if a heart was cooled until it stopped beating, it could be restarted using an electrical pacemaker. This led to his invention of the world's first heart pacemaker in 1950.

Hopps' machine was bulky – measuring about 30cm/1ft long and a few centimetres wide and deep. But with the invention of transistors and more reliable batteries smaller versions were developed.

In 1957 an engineer from Minneapolis called Earl Bakken produced the first external pacemaker. It was in a small box with controls that allowed the heart rate and the strength of the voltage to be adjusted manually. The box was connected to electrode leads that passed through the skin ending in the heart muscle.

The first completely internal pacemaker was inserted into Arne Larsson in 1958 at the Karolinska University Hospital in Solna, Sweden, using a pacemaker designed by Rune Elmqvist and surgeon Åke Senning. It was connected to electrodes that were attached to the heart muscle during open heart surgery. This pacemaker only lasted three hours and a second device lasted two days. Larsson went on to have 22 different pacemakers before he died in 2001.

The Link Between Smoking and Lung Cancer

Austin Bradford Hill (1897–1991)
Richard Doll (1912–2005)

In 1900 when smoking jackets and after dinner cigars were the height of fashion, few people were concerned about the health risks. And nobody wanted to hear what we now know about the link with cancer and other diseases.

During the First and Second World Wars (1914–1918 and 1939–1945 respectively), when millions died, the extra deaths from smoking related diseases went unnoticed. However, soon after the war, lung cancer seemed to be a more obvious problem, and led to interest from the Medical Research Council where Richard Doll was working for the Statistical Research Unit and Austin Hill was a statistician.

In 1947 the two men began working together to analyze the possible causes of lung cancer. Their statistical survey was published in 1951, and was the result of interviews with 700 patients from 20 London hospitals. Doll said later that it became so clear early that smoking was a factor that he gave up the habit himself halfway through the research.

This initial research was published in 1951, by which time they had started another study – asking 40,000 doctors if they smoked. They compared these answers with information about doctors who went on to develop lung cancer, and found a direct link. When the health minister for the United Kingdom, Iain Macleod (1913–1970), called a news conference to announce the findings in 1954, he said:

It must be regarded as established that there is a relationship between smoking and cancer of the lung.

Macleod chain-smoked throughout the announcement.

When Doll moved to Oxford University in 1969, he continued to follow up the initial group of doctors. In the 20, 40 and 50-year follow up studies Doll – now working with Richard Peto, professor of epidermiology and medical statistics at the University of Oxford, (b. 1943) – showed conclusively that smokers were far more likely to die not only from lung cancer but also from other smoking related diseases like heart disease, and tongue and throat cancer. They also showed that quitting cut the risks. As a result of this research, many millions of people have given up smoking, avoiding premature death.

Smoking is now banned in all enclosed public spaces.

Antipsychotics

Henri Laborit (1914–1995)

In the mid-20th century, new developments in pharmacology led to the introduction of medicines that could influence the treatment of profoundly disturbed psychiatric patients. This marked a change in the history of mental illness, providing an alternative to locking people away in asylums.

Before this time schizophrenics were considered untreatable and interned in mental hospitals often for many years. Restraints were commonplace, and patients had little hope of recovery. For the first time there was now an alternative treatment and patients could be released into the community to lead a normal life.

The first drug of this kind was discovered almost by accident. Henri Laborit, a French naval surgeon, was experimenting with different cocktails of medicines to anaesthetize his patients. At the same time, Paul Charpentier – a chemist working for the chemical group Rhône-Poulenc – produced a new drug called chlorpromazine. When Laborit introduced it into his mixture of drugs he found it produced a change in the patient's mood, which he called a 'pharmacological lobotomy'. Patients were sedated with no anxiety or pain, but were not asleep.

Laborit's work came to the attention of two psychiatrists, Jean Delay and Pierre Deniker, working at the psychiatric hospital Sainte Anne in Paris. They used chlorpromazine on its own by daily injection, and found that patients with delusions and hallucinations typical of schizophrenia improved dramatically.

As a result, from 1956, the numbers of inmates in psychiatric asylums began to fall dramatically.

The Structure of DNA

James Watson (b. 1928)
Francis Crick (1916–2004)

James Watson's and Francis Crick's ground-breaking research demonstrated the double helix, twisted ladder, structure of DNA (deoxyribonucleic acid) and that DNA was involved in the transmission of inheritance.

By the 1920s it was already known that the nucleus of every cell contained two types of nucleic acid: RNA (ribonucleic acid) and DNA and that these were involved in the process of inheritance. However, it wasn't until Watson and Crick's significant work highlighted the complicated structure of DNA that scientists realized that it contained the complete code for life.

The double helix of DNA is made up of two chains of alternating sugar and phosphate groups. Four types of chemical, known as bases, form the rungs of the 'ladder' of the double helix. These are adenine (A), cytosine (C), guanine (G), and thymine (T). They can only be linked in certain combination, A, links with T, and C with G, T with A, and G with C. The way in which these pairs of bases are arranged determines the characteristics of a human being.

Watson and Crick were awarded the 1962 Nobel Prize for physiology or medicine along with British biophysicist Maurice Wilkins (1916–2004), whose X-ray diffraction studies of DNA had proved crucial to their determination of DNA's molecular structure. Watson and Crick's work in this field marked the birth of genetics.

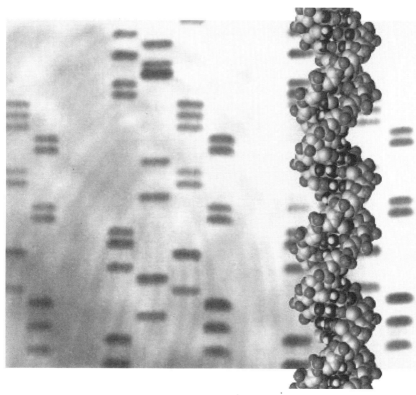

The molecular structure of DNA.

See: *Preimplantation Genetic Diagnosis,* pages 196–197;
Human Genome Project, pages 207–208

Heart–Lung Machine

John Gibbon (1903–1973)

The heart–lung machine is designed to perform the functions of both the lungs and heart of a patient during surgery.

The patient's blood is diverted into the machine where it is oxygenated and pumped around the body. Suspending the normal function of the heart and lungs for the duration of the operation allows the surgeon to operate on heart defects. The invention of the heart–lung machine paved the way for the modern era in cardiac surgery.

Before this invention, there were many operations on the heart that were not possible while the heart was beating. Interrupting the blood supply for more than four minutes results in brain damage, but most procedures are too complex to be undertaken in this time frame.

The new invention was first used successfully on 18-year-old Cecilia Bavolek, who had a hole in her heart. On 6 May 1953 she was connected to the heart-lung machine for 45 minutes while the repair was carried out.

Although John Gibbon is credited with making the first heart–lung machine, Willem Kolff (b. 1911) had already done much of the preparatory work. Kolff was a Dutch physician working in America. In 1955 he designed a pump made from disposable polyethylene tubing that oxygenated the blood. He was already famous for inventing the first dialysis machine in 1943 but, unfortunately, he failed to patent his pump oxygenator.

The Placebo Effect

Henry Knowles Beecher (1904–1976)

The mind has a powerful effect on healing, pain control and general well being, which still isn't fully understood. The placebo effect highlights this.

In 1955, Henry K. Beecher, an anaesthetist working at Massachusetts General Hospital, reported on the so-called placebo effect and published the classic work *The Powerful Placebo*.

Beecher claimed that, in about 35 per cent of cases, patients who took a pill containing no active ingredients experienced an improvement in their condition.

One possible explanation is that the process of believing in a treatment could actually have an effect on the chemical reactions in the brain. This might in turn influence the rest of the body, including the immune system. This forms the basis for the belief that positive thinking can bring about healing.

An alternative explanation is that the placebo effect is the result of a change in behaviour. As children we learn to behave in a certain way when we feel ill. Believing a treatment is working will bring about a change in behaviour. This includes a change in attitude and this may in turn affect brain biochemistry.

Beecher's work was followed by the foundation of The American Society of Psychosomatic Medicine, which further explored the placebo effect.

Polio Vaccine

Jonas Salk (1914–1995)
Albert Sabin (1906–1993)

Widespread outbreaks of polio causing crippling disabilities or deaths were virtually eliminated with the introduction of polio immunization in the 1950s.

In the late 19th century many lives were affected by polio. Despite successes with other vaccines, it proved hard to develop one against polio.

Five years after US President Franklin Delano Roosevelt (1882–1945) – himself a victim of polio – came to power in 1932, he set up the National Foundation for Infantile Paralysis. This provided the financial incentive researchers needed to find a solution.

In 1947 Jonas Salk was appointed at the National Foundation as head of the research team looking into virus infections. He began experimenting with injecting dead polio virus into previously infected children and in 1952 he found that this stimulated the production of antibodies against the virus.

Salk then injected the vaccine into healthy volunteers including his wife and children. All the volunteers developed antibodies to polio, and none developed the disease. Impressed by these results, the United States administration began to implement a programme of vaccination and by 1955 over four million people had received the vaccine.

At the same time, Albert Sabin was working in Cincinnati Children's Hospital where he was head of research. He developed a similar vaccine to Salk's using weak strains of the poliovirus. This was taken by mouth on a sugar lump (to disguise the taste) and not by injection. Being cheaper than the injection, Sabin's vaccine has been used more widely since its introduction in 1957 and has become the main defense against polio throughout the world.

Bone Marrow Transplant

E. Donnall Thomas (b. 1920)

Before bone marrow transplants, patients with leukaemia had little hope of survival. This discovery improved their survival rates dramatically.

Bone marrow contains blood-forming cells, known as stem cells, which make red blood cells to carry oxygen, white blood cells to fight infections, and platelets which stem bleeding.

Diseases interfering with the production of any of these cells include cancers, such as leukaemia and lymphomas, and also non-cancerous conditions such as inherited disorders of the immune system that affect white cell production, as well as aplastic anaemia – a condition affecting red cell production.

A bone marrow transplant treats patients with high-dose chemotherapy or radiation, killing all the cells in the bone marrow including the diseased ones, and then replacing damaged marrow with marrow from a healthy donor.

Donnall Thomas, a physician from Seattle, carried out the first successful bone marrow transplant in 1956, giving a leukaemia patient healthy bone marrow from his identical twin. The patient's body accepted the donated bone marrow and used it to make new healthy red and white blood cells and platelets.

Thomas realized the importance of matching the donor and the recipient as closely as possible because when the bone marrow is transplanted, the recipient's immune system recognizes it as foreign and attacks it. Also, the cells of the donor bone marrow can actually attack the recipient's tissue, a problem known as 'graft versus host disease'.

Thomas and his team were closely involved in developing drugs to overcome these problems, which enabled him in 1969 to carry out the first successful bone marrow transplant from a relative who was not an identical twin to a patient with leukaemia.

Ultrasound

Ian Donald (1910–1987)

*Being able to see the growing foetus
inside the woman's womb is a relatively recent
breakthrough in medical history.*

Ultrasound was invented in 1957 by Ian Donald, an obstetrician and gynaecologist working in Scotland, and was used for the first time on pregnant women in 1958.

The technology relies on very high frequency sound waves that penetrate the body without causing it any harm. When the waves encounter an internal organ such as a bone or muscle they bounce back. The reflected waves look different depending on what they have hit inside the body. A monitor detects the reflected waves and can be used to identify the shape, size and consistency of the internal organs.

Ultrasound technology grew out of research into radar and sonar developed in the early 20th century. Donald became familiar with their use in identifying submarines when he served with the RAF during the Second World War (1939–45).

He was known in some circles as 'Mad Donald' because of his passion for gadgets, which he described as a 'childish interest in machines, electronic and otherwise.' Convinced that sonar could somehow be used for medical diagnosis, he started to make further investigations.

In 1955 Donald visited the research department of the boilermakers Babcock & Wilcox at Renfrew, near Glasgow, where he carried out experiments using their ultrasonic metal-flaw detector. He used the machine to examine the image produced by pathological specimens that he had removed during surgical procedures, including fibroids and ovarian cysts, and compared them with a piece of steak which he used as his control measure, being similar in consistency to ovarian tissue and the muscular tissue of fibroids.

Hearing about Donald's work, the physicist Thomas Brown, of the engineering firm Kelvin and Hughes Scientific Instruments Company, rang and offered his help. Brown and Donald teamed up with John MacVicar, a junior doctor in Donald's department, to invent the world's first ultrasound scanner. It had a transducer which could be moved over the patient's abdomen and produced a two-dimensional image on a monitor.

Results of their research first appeared in *The Lancet* in 1958 under the title *Investigation of Abdominal Masses by Pulsed Ultrasound*. There was some initial scepticism from their colleagues, which soon dissolved once they realized the potential that it presented. Notably, Donald presented the case of a woman with an ovarian cyst that had previously been diagnosed as ovarian cancer. It was therefore possible to see how the new technology could make a difference to diagnosis and treatment. As Donald said:

> *'As soon as we got rid of the backroom attitude and brought our apparatus fully into the Department with an inexhaustible supply of living patients with fascinating clinical problems, we were able to get ahead really fast.'*

As it gained in followers, the early design was updated and improved, and then in 1960 it began commercial production as the 'Diasonograph'.

Donald was awarded the CBE in 1973 in recognition of his contribution to medical science.

Levodopa for Parkinson's Disease

Arvid Carlsson (b. 1923)

Studies in the mid-20th century led to the discovery that levodopa could relieve the symptoms of patients suffering the effects of Parkinson's disease.

In 1817 British physician James Parkinson first described the 'shaking palsy', in which patients often have an uncontrollable tremor. This is known today as Parkinson's Disease. Patients also typically have stiff movements and an impassive expression. It is a degenerative condition and famous sufferers include boxer Mohammed Ali (b. 1942), actor Michael J. Fox (b. 1961) and the late Pope John Paul II (1920–2005).

Until the introduction of levodopa (or L-dopa) there was little that doctors could do to help patients with this condition. Then in 1957, Arvid Carlsson, a Swedish professor of Medicine, found that the chemical dopamine was involved in the transmission of nerve impulses in the brain. He then developed a method for measuring the dopamine in brain tissues and found that it was largely concentrated in an area of the brain called the basal ganglia that is important in the control of movement.

Carlsson went on to show that giving animals a drug called reserpine resulted in a fall in the level of dopamine. The animals then found it difficult to control movements normally, similar to the symptoms of Parkinson's disease. When given levodopa, the animals' symptoms improved.

We now know that the brain contains several areas involved in the normal control of movement, including the substantia nigra, the cerebellum and the basal ganglia. They are connected via nerves and dopamine is important in the transmission of information along these nerves. In Parkinson's disease there is a fall in the amount of dopamine in the substantia nigra. Originally isolated from vicia faba beans in 1911 and thought to be biologically inactive, levodopa works by being converted to dopamine in the brain, and therefore relieving the symptoms.

After Carlsson's discovery, doctors began to give levodopa tentatively, but results were disappointing. In 1967 George Cotzias (1918–1977), a neurologist working at Cornell Medical Centre in New York, began giving larger doses over longer periods of time and had correspondingly better results.

One of the most dramatic effects of levodopa came in 1969, when British-born neurologist Oliver Sacks, working in Beth Abraham Hospital in the Bronx, New York, used it to treat patients affected by the 1917–1928 epidemic of *encephalitis lethargica*. These patients had not been able to move or speak for years and were suffering from a severe form of Parkinson's disease. Their response to the drug was dramatized in the 1990 film *Awakenings* based on Sacks' 1973 book of the same name.

In 2000, Carlsson won the Nobel Prize in Physiology or Medicine for his contribution to medicine.

Foetal Monitoring

Orvan Hess (1906–2002)
Edward Hon (1917–2001)

The cardiotocograph is a machine invented in 1957 by two obstetricians and gynaecologists to allow the baby's heart rate to be monitored in labour.

Before inventing this machine with Edward Hon, Orvan Hess described childbirth as a 'watch-and-wait-and-pray' experience, because there was no way of finding out about the baby's state of health other than by listening with a Pinard stethoscope between contractions. During the contractions, when the baby is most likely to get into difficulty maintaining its own blood supply, it was previously not possible to hear the baby's heartbeat at all.

Hess and Hon's first machine designed to monitor the baby's heart rate electronically was bulky, at over six-feet-tall. Advances in technology have brought the size down to a much smaller bedside machine, which is still widely used in the labour room to measure both the baby's heart rate and the mother's contractions.

Most machines use two discs placed on the mother's abdomen and held in place with elasticated belts. Wires attach the discs to the machine, which shows the uterus contractions and foetal heart rate on a monitor, and can be printed out on paper.

Since the 1960s, the cardiotocograph has been used widely in delivery rooms all over the world. However, since its introduction there has been some debate about its value. The monitoring is supposed to identify a baby in distress in the womb, but several research studies have suggested that it is no better at doing this than periodically checking the foetal heartbeat with a Pinard stethoscope.

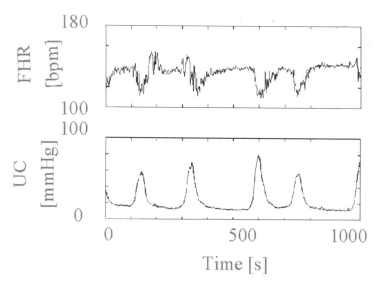

The above shows a typical foetal monitoring readout showing the foetal heart rate (FHR) in beats per minute (bpm) on the upper trace and uterine contractions (UC) in millimetres of mercury (mmHg, the units of pressure) on the lower trace.

See: *Pinard Stethoscope,* page 75

The Eradication of Smallpox

The eradication of smallpox has saved an estimated 1.5 million lives a year since the last case in 1977. There have also been massive financial savings as vaccine, medical care and quarantine facilities are no longer required.

There is no cure for smallpox. A third of people infected with the disease die as a result, and those that survive are scarred for life, with deep pockmarks all over their body, and often blinded.

Smallpox was no respecter of class or status, its more prominent victims included Queen Mary II of England, Emperor Joseph I of Austria, King Luis I of Spain, Tsar Peter II of Russia, Queen Ulkrika Elenora of Sweden and King Louis XV of France.

In the 1950s, there was no systematic global programme for vaccination and millions of people died from smallpox every year. During this period, the use of available vaccines was largely confined to certain groups in industrialized countries. For instance, smallpox vaccine was offered to all age groups, but only those at risk – health care workers and travellers – were specially targeted. This policy meant that many people remained unprotected, and outbreaks continued to occur. During an outbreak the health authorities mounted massive vaccination programmes combined with isolation or quarantine of infected individuals or suspected cases.

The first attempt to introduce a more cohesive vaccination programme began in 1958 when the World Health Organization (WHO) decided to eradicate smallpox worldwide. The disease was chosen for eradication because the vaccine was both highly effective and affordable. It also helped that smallpox is easy to diagnose without the need for any laboratory tests.

The whole world was involved in the vaccination programme. In the late 1960s, the WHO added an additional strategy identifying any smallpox cases and quarantining them. All contacts with that person were then located and vaccinated.

Hip Replacement

John Charnley (1911–1982)

The elderly often have weakened bones which are more likely to break after a fall. The hip joint is particularly vulnerable.

With advances in surgery, infection control and engineering, it is now possible to replace completely the broken joint with an artificial one. The same technique can be used to replace hips in elderly people with severe arthritis.

Before the advent of hip replacement surgery there was no treatment for a broken hip. Sometimes patients were put in traction or a small plaster of paris cast. However, they were prone to complications, such as pneumonia and urinary tract infections, and about half of those over the age of 60 died as a result.

The first attempts at hip surgery involved trying to remove irregular lumps of bone and cartilage from deformed and misshapen arthritic joints. Gradually surgeons began to experiment with different materials for resurfacing the ball of the hip joint. One of the first was M. N. Smith-Peterson, (1886–1953) an orthopaedic surgeon from Boston, Massachusetts. In 1925 he made a hollow hemispherical glass mould which could fit over the ball of the hip joint and provide a new smooth surface. The glass wasn't rejected by the immune system but failed because it couldn't withstand the stress of walking. During the 1930s and 1940s he and others experimented with plastic and stainless steel and other metals, which were stronger and didn't corrode.

But although the materials improved, the technique still needed development. The implants tended to loosen as a result of friction and were no use for patients who had deformities affecting the socket (acetabulum) of the hip joint as well as the ball (femoral head).

In the 1940s, the French surgeon Jean Judet (1905–1995) heard from an Ear, Nose and Throat specialist about a glue called methyl methacrylate, which he was using to reconstruct the orbit and nose. Judet realized that this glue might be useful in orthopaedic surgery. Using acrylic to make artificial replacements for the ball of the joint he designed a ball with a stem that could glued into the shaft of the leg bone. The first implanted hip was inserted in 1946 in a wine merchant from Boulogne – disabled with hip arthritis. He was up and about, drinking wine, a week after the surgery.

The second patient was an elderly lady with a fractured hip who also had a successful outcome. News spread and it became very popular. However, although these glued-in hip replacements were a great improvement, they still tended to fail after three or four years, often as a result of damage to the socket.

In England John Charnley was attempting to solve the problems affecting hip surgery. In 1958, he became the first surgeon to solve the problem of the eroding acetabulum by replacing it with an implant at the same time as replacing the femoral head. He cut off the upper part of the femur, replacing it

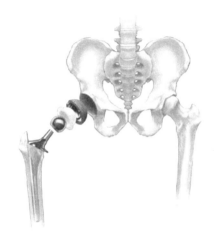

*A typical hip replacement includes (*from left to right*) a femoral stem, a bearing, a liner, and an acetabular cap.*

with a metal ball on a metal stem, which was pushed and then glued into the remaining bone. Then, using polymethyl methacrylate cement, he glued a polyethylene liner in a metal shell into a hollowed out area of the acetabulum. When he pushed the metal ball into the liner, the ball snapped into place and this was the first total hip replacement.

Charnley followed up his patients closely. He wrote to them all asking if he could have their hips back when they died and because most of them were so pleased with their hip, they agreed!

The Structure of Antibodies

Gerald Edelman (USA b.1929)
Rodney Porter (UK (1917–1985)

Antibodies are an important part of the body's defence system.

Discovering the chemical structure of antibodies has enabled scientists to gain a better knowledge and understanding of immunity and is considered an important breakthrough in medical history.

We know now that antibodies, (also known as immunoglobulins) are made by the white blood cells in the immune system to neutralize foreign invaders (also called antigens) into the body, such as viruses and bacteria. They do this by binding tightly to the antigen, thereby marking them out for other parts of the immune system to destroy.

Gerald Edelman, an American biologist, and Rodney Porter, an English biochemist, were working independently in different countries in the 1950s. But their work, as a whole, clearly described the structure of antibodies for the first time, as four chains of protein bound together in the shape of the letter Y. Following their breakthrough discovery, researchers went on to discover the five main types of antibodies: IgA (Immunoglobulin A), IgD, IgE, IgG and IgM.

The body is capable of making millions of different subtypes of antibody, all slightly different, in response to the many infectious threats. The V-shaped part of the antibody chain attaches to potentially threatening foreign objects (antigens) to destroy them.

Edelman and Porter were awarded the 1972 Nobel Prize for Physiology or Medicine in recognition of their pioneering work.

Oral Rehydration Fluid

The discovery of oral rehydration fluid, a simple solution of glucose and minerals, has done more to prevent deaths from diarrhoea than any other medical intervention.

More than 150 years ago doctors established that patients suffering from diarrhoea and vomiting lose both water and mineral salts, including sodium, potassium and chloride. In the 1960s, doctors treating cholera in Vietnam, Calcutta, India and Dhakha, Bangladesh began to use this knowledge to provide dehydrated patients with drinks of water, mixed with glucose and the other minerals as an alternative to an intravenous drip of the same solution.

This seemed to work, but their experience was not enough to convince the World Health Organization (WHO), who still argued that intravenous fluid was the preferred treatment for dehydration.

The opportunity for a breakthrough came in 1971, when the Bangladesh war of independence led to an estimated 10 million people moving into refugee camps in West Bengal. There was a cholera epidemic and the West Bengal government didn't have enough resources to keep up with the requirement for intravenous fluid replacement, partly because this treatment needed to be administered by medical professionals who were simply overwhelmed by the numbers of people needing help. The situation was desperate and thousands of people were dying daily.

In one of the health centres in the camp, Dilip Mahalanabis was familiar with oral rehydration fluid from his medical training in Calcutta. He decided to try the same thing in the refugee camp.

At the time, oral rehydration fluid was only supposed to be given out by health professionals. However, Mahalanabis gave it out in dried form to patients and families to reconstitute with water and distribute to the sick.

He instructed them to drink large volumes of the solution in the early stages of their illness.

Where previously doctors had spent most of their time giving out oral rehydration fluid or inserting intravenous drips, Mahalanabis' method freed up the medical professionals to concentrate on refilling the supply of oral rehydration fluid and making short visits to the sick. His efforts were a success and, as a result, the death rate in his camp fell to about 3 per cent in 2 months compared with nearly 10 times that in the other camps.

Later the same year, Dhiman Barua, head of the Bacterial Diseases Unit of the WHO, visited the camp, and was impressed by Mahalanabis' efforts. Despite scepticism from other doctors, Barua created the WHO's diarrhoeal disease-control programme in 1978, supporting the treatment of diarrhoea with oral rehydration fluid, and only giving intravenous fluid if that failed.

As a result of this programme, the number of children under five dying each year from diarrhoea has dropped from nearly 5 million in the 1980s to 1.8 million in 2000. Nonetheless, this is still a horrifying statistic, and many more children could be saved if they had access to clean water and basic medical treatment.

Glue for Wounds

Harry Coover (b. 1919)

When Super Glue® was first invented, its medical uses were overlooked. Now it has become standard practice to use a version of it to close the edges of small wounds, particularly in children, instead of using stitches or paper strips.

The chemist, Harry Coover originally developed superglue in 1942 while working for Eastman Kodak Company and searching for a clear plastic to use to make gunsight lenses. The cyanoacrylate compound he made was rejected because it was too sticky.

It wasn't until nearly 20 years later that Coover realised that cyanoacrylate might be useful as commercial glue, and in the early 1960s Eastman Kodak began working with Ethicon – a company famous for producing medical sutures – to research the medical uses of cyanoacrylate.

A spray version of the glue was used in Vietnam to treat wounded service personnel. On the battlefield, uncontrolled bleeding is a significant cause of mortality, and there has always been a keen interest in developing new treatments.

Describing the spray's use, Coover said:

'If somebody had a chest wound or open wound that was bleeding, the biggest problem they had was stopping the bleeding so they could get the patient back to the hospital. And the consequence was – many of them bled to death. So the medics used the spray, stopped the bleeding, and were able to get the wounded back to the base hospital. And many, many lives were saved.'

It was some years before the glue was approved for more general medical use. The delay was partly because the original compound tended to cause skin irritation. By the 1970s, however, scientists had developed a less irritating version known as N-butyl-2-cyanoacrylate, which was used extensively in Canada.

A compound called 2-octylcyanoacrylate is the latest in cyanoacrylate technology. It is almost four times as strong as N-butyl-2-cyanoacrylate and reaches maximum bonding strength in less than three minutes, at which point it is equivalent in strength to healed tissue at seven days post repair.

Used widely for treating small wounds that close easily without any tension, the glue is particularly useful for treating children. Unlike stitches, which need a local anaesthetic first, administered with a needle, glue can be applied directly to the wound after it has been cleaned. There are no stitches to remove a week later, and there is much less risk of scarring.

Cognitive Behavioural Therapy (CBT)

Aaron Temkin Beck (b.1921)

CBT is a popular talking therapy for a variety of psychological conditions, including anxiety, anger, panic and depression.

CBT is based on the principle that if your thinking is distorted, your emotions will follow. Therefore, understanding and then changing your thinking will have an impact on how you feel. Likewise, improved behaviour will have an educational effect on the thought processing, reinforcing positive thinking.

The idea of CBT goes back to the 1st century Greek philosopher Epictetus (AD 55–135), who wrote: *'Men are disturbed not by things, but by the view which they take of them.'*

The work of Albert Ellis (1913–2007), an American psychoanalyst, was also a powerful influence in the development of this theory. He described a similar one in the 1950s that he called Rational Emotive Behaviour Therapy, as a direct response to his dislike of the non-directive nature of psychoanalysis. His approach required the therapist to be more involved in helping the client to adjust unhelpful thinking patterns – which is a central part of CBT.

Most people regard American psychiatrist and psychoanalyst Aaron Beck as the driving force behind cognitive therapy. Beck's theory is founded on the belief that people are not passive recipients of outside forces, but have the power to change their lives and that they are able to do this throughout their lives. He believed that people are constantly attributing emotional as well as intellectual significance to daily events, not always helpfully, and that the way each person does this reflects his or her personality.

The purpose of the therapy is to question habitually unhelpful ways of interpreting information, by first learning to recognize them with the help of the therapist. This is achieved by discussion with the therapist, and a series of homework tasks, such as keeping a diary of thoughts and emotions in particular situations. Then the client learns new, more constructive ways of providing meaning.

One way of doing this is to look at the diary of thoughts, and to consider if there are any alternative, more positive ways of thinking about a situation. If so, what might be the resulting feeling associated with the new thought.

The idea is to teach the client to challenge their own negative thoughts, so that they can experience the more positive emotion that results from positive, constructive thinking.

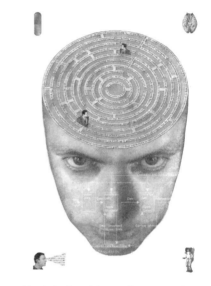

Cognitive behavioural therapy focusses on the way in which our brains represent and process knowledge.

The Contraceptive Pill

Gregory Pinkus (1903–1967)
Carl Djerassi (b.1923)

Developed in the 1950s, the pill works by suppressing ovulation. Its introduction has revolutionized contraception, sexual behaviour and women's reproductive rights.

In the 1950s Gregory Pinkus was a biologist struggling to make a living as a visiting professor researching steroids at Clarke University, Worcester, Massachusetts, while moonlighting as a lab caretaker to make ends meet. However, from the moment he met Margaret Sanger (1879–1966), the course of his life was to change forever.

Sanger was a birth-control activist, already in her 70s by the time she met Pinkus at a dinner party. At this time in America, there were restrictions on the sale and use of birth control in 30 of the 52 US states. Sanger, motivated by seeing her own mother go through eighteen pregnancies and eleven live births, dreamt of a future when inexpensive birth control would be universally available.

She believed it was possible to develop a birth-control pill, as easy to take as aspirin. However the United States government, medical institutions and the pharmaceutical industry wanted nothing to do with contraceptive research and progress was slow.

When Sanger met Pinkus she realized that he might have the knowledge to be able to develop her dream. In 1953, she introduced him to her friend Margaret McCormack (1875–1967), a well-known American philanthropist. McCormack had studied biology, graduating in 1904, but had given up a career when she got married, normal practice at the time. She supported Sanger's cause and was enthusiastic about the possibility of a birth-control pill.

Thanks to McCormack's generous financial support, Pinkus and his colleague, Min-Chueh Chang (1908–1991), started work using a steroid called progesterone just discovered by Carl Djerassi, a chemist working in New Mexico. They proved that repeated injections of progesterone stopped ovulation in animals.

Meanwhile, McCormack followed the research closely and pushed for quicker results. She was, by all accounts, a formidable woman, nearly 1.83m/6ft tall, and was described by Mrs Pinkus as a warrior: '... *she carried herself like a ramrod. Little old woman she was not. She was a grenadier.*'

Pinkus's challenge was to find something as good as the progesterone injections, but in tablet form. He began collaborating with John Rock (1890–1984), a fertility specialist to give synthetically produced progesterone tablets to small groups of volunteers. Encouraged by their results, in 1956 they launched large-scale trials in Haiti and Puerto Rico, giving women a pill containing synthetic versions of the hormones oestrogen and progesterone.

Their pill worked, and by 1960 the drug was approvedand launched. Pinkus received international acclaim and the pill became popular overnight. In the United States around 1.2 million women used the pill within two years of its launch. When it was introduced in the United Kingdom in 1961, initially it was for married women only, but that changed by 1967. It has continued to be one of the most popular forms of contraception in the United Kingdom.

Although there have been a few health scares about the pill since its introduction, the dose of hormones is now much lower than in the pills introduced in the 1960s, and doctors believe that for healthy, non-smoking women it is relatively safe. It is also known to protect against cancer of the ovaries and the womb lining and also pelvic inflammatory disease – a common cause of infertility.

Few men think much about how the pill affects them. However, chemistry professor Carl Djerassi, leader of the research team that synthesized the first steroid oral contraceptive on 15 October 1951, wrote an entire book on how the pill has touched his life.

The First Artificial Heart Valve

Nina Starr-Braunwald (1928–1992)

Dr Nina Starr-Braunwald designed the valve and then led the surgical team that implanted it.

There are four valves in the heart that regulate the flow of blood between the four chambers. In the early 20th century, valve disease was common, often the result of rheumatic fever.

Those that did not die from the disease suffered as a result of damage to the heart valves, which leaked or didn't open fully, or both. There were also many people suffering the results of congenital heart valve disease and other degenerative valve disorders, none of whom could expect a cure.

Surgery to replace or repair heart valves only became possible because of the advances in general anaesthesia, and the invention of the heart lung machine – an extraordinary discovery which was designed to perform the functions of both the lungs and heart of a patient during the procedure. It allowed surgeons to operate on the heart which was cooled until it stopped beating, while the machine continued to pump blood around the body. At the end of the operation the heart was warmed up until it started beating again.

Nina Starr-Braunwald was one of the first female general surgeons at New York's Bellvue Hospital. She was interested in research into prosthetic heart valves, and developed one made of a flexible polyurethane and Teflon material that she implanted successfully into dogs.

In early 1960 she moved from dogs to people, and the first person to receive the valve did well for several months.

Although Starr-Braunwald was the first, two other surgeons achieved similar success the same year and are often quoted as the inventors of the prosthetic heart valve. First was Dwight Harken

(1910–1993), a Boston surgeon who developed a valve designed like a ball and cage. Two of his seven patients survived the procedure. Later the same year, Portland surgeon Albert Starr and retired engineer Lowell Edwards invented a slightly different ball and cage design prosthetic valve with six of the first eight patients surviving. In fact, the valve was so successful that the first man to receive the Starr-Edwards valve lived for 10 years and only died when he fell off a ladder.

The Starr-Edwards valve became very popular, partly because Edwards set up Edwards Laboratories and began to produce it commercially.

Over the years, there have been many modifications in design, and the operation has become so common that now there are around 300,000 people in the world receiving prosthetic heart valves every year.

See: *General Anaesthetic,* pages 48–49; *Heart–Lung Machine*, page 131

Methadone Treatment

Vincent Dole (1913–2006)
Marie Nyswander (1919–1986)
Mary Jeanne Kreek (b. 1913)

The introduction of methadone as a treatment for heroin addicts marked a significant change in the perception of addiction. Before then little was understood about the biology of the condition, and there was no medical treatment.

Although the euphoric effects of heroin have been known about since 3000 BC, it was not until the 19th century that it became associated with criminal behaviour and social outcasts. Until the 1960s little was understood about the biological nature of addiction, and many addicts were put in prison with no treatment.

Vincent Dole, a physician at Rockefeller University in New York wanted to understand more about addiction. One of the few books available on the subject was written by Marie Nyswander, a psychiatrist running a street clinic for addicts in New York, who later became Dole's second wife. In her book *The Drug Addict as a Patient*, published in 1956, she argued that heroin addiction was a medical problem.

If Nyswander was correct, Dole believed that addiction could potentially be treated just like any other chronic condition – such as diabetes or heart disease.

He set up a research project to investigate possible drug treatments, recruiting Nyswander and a researcher – Mary Jeanne Kreek – to help him. Addicts from Nyswander's clinic volunteered to be admitted to hospital and given different drug treatments for their

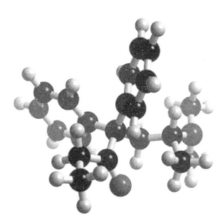

The molecular structure of methadone.

addiction. Rapidly it became clear that methadone might be useful.

Methadone was already being used as a pain reliever and cough suppressant. It was developed during the Second World War (1939–1945) as an alternative to morphine. The research project showed that treatment with methadone enabled drug addicts to lead a more normal life. It works by preventing the withdrawal symptons and cravings associated with heroin. And because it can be taken by mouth in liquid form, rather than by injection, there is less risk of disease transmission or accidental overdose.

In the last 10 years, Buprenorphine (Subutex) has overtaken methadone as a better treatment for recovering addicts. However, at the time, the work done by Dole, Nyswander and Kreek had a groundbreaking effect on shifting the perception of heroin addiction into a medically treatable condition.

Angioplasty

Melvin P. Judkins (1922–1985)
Charles Dotter (1920–1985)

Before angioplasty was invented, patients with blocked or narrowed coronary arteries were offered open-heart surgery and coronary-artery bypass grafts.

Patients were admitted to hospital, often for a week or more, and left with a scar on the chest and another the length of one leg. With the advent of angioplasty, most patients can now have the same result after a minimally invasive outpatient procedure, with far less discomfort.

Melvin Judkins invented angioplasty in collaboration with Charles Theodore Dotter, both working as radiologists in Portland in the 1960s. Together they pioneered new techniques in radiology that helped to move their specialty away from working largely on the interpretation of images in a darkened room, and into a more highly specialized field where doctors can combine minimally invasive surgery with high-resolution imaging.

Angioplasty is one step on from angiography – first carried out in 1949, to investigate the arterial circulation of the organs. The procedure involves the insertion of a thin flexible tube, or catheter, into an artery. The radiologist gently threads the catheter through to the artery that needs studying. Then a dye is injected which looks opaque on an X-ray. Therefore, where blood flows easily it appears opaque, and where it does not, nothing will show.

In 1964 Dotter and Judkins realized that it was possible to open any blockage seen on a coronary artery angiogram by inserting a narrow catheter into the suspect artery itself. They called this technique 'angioplasty'.

In 1967 Judkins devised a system for shaping a wire to match closely the

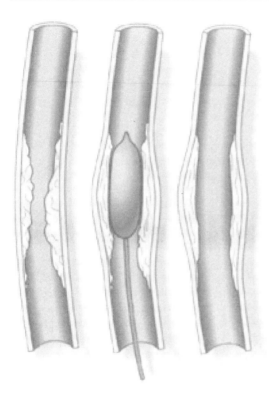

An artery before, during and after balloon angioplasty. Images from left to right show: the narrowed portion of the artery; a catheter inserted and the balloon inflated inside the narrowed artery; the artery no longer narrowed after the procedure.

patient's coronary artery as seen on an angiogram. The catheter was placed over the wire and then both were heated in boiling water. Once they had both cooled down, the wire was removed and the catheter retained the shape of the wire. Judkins' coronary catheters became commercially available a year later.

A German cardiologist, Andreas Gruentzig (1939–1985), refashioned the design of the catheter in 1975, to include a balloon which could be inflated when the catheter is in position inside the coronary artery that is narrowed or blocked. His first successful cases in 1977 met with resounding support from his colleagues, and balloon angioplasty has been widely used ever since.

Contraceptive Implant

Sheldon Jerome Segal (b. 1926)
Horacio B. Croxatto

The idea that women could prevent pregnancy simply by having an implant under the skin has been a breakthrough in modern contraceptive technology.

The implant releases a steady stream of the hormone progesterone that flows around the woman's bloodstream to her reproductive organs. This prevents ovulation and stops the sperm from getting through the cervix into the womb.

Sheldon Segal originally had the idea for this innovation in 1965 when he was head of the Population Council's biomedical research staff. His idea was to use capsules made of silastic, a polymerized silicone rubber used in surgical tubing, pacemakers, and prosthetic devices because it is well tolerated by the body.

Horacio Croxatto a Chilean physician, who then became a Fellow at the Population Council, developed the delivery system by creating the capsule.

Nearly 20 years of clinical trials followed, and finally in 1983 the first contraceptive implant was approved – initially in Finland, with other countries following suit. It was called Norplant and consisted of six flexible rods, each about the length of a match. A specially trained doctor inserted the rods under the skin on the inner upper arm. Each rod contained levonorgestrel, a synthetic form of the natural female hormone progesterone, and the implant provided contraceptive cover for five years.

However, Norplant proved to be difficult to remove, and in 1999 it was discontinued in favour of a single rod implant: Implanon, containing a similar progesterone hormone called etonorgestrel.

Coronary–Artery Bypass Grafting

René Gerónimo Favaloro (1923–2000)

Learning how to bypass an artery that is in danger of blocking completely by using a vein graft has transformed cardiology, and millions of patients have benefited from coronary artery bypass grafts (CABG) since its introduction.

The coronary arteries supply oxygen to the heart muscle. With age, all the body's arteries become harder and narrower, a process known as atherosclerosis. This is accelerated by age, smoking, diabetes and a high-fat diet.

When it occurs in the coronary arteries it is known as Coronary Artery Disease and can cause chest pain, or angina, or a heart attack. A complete blockage in one or more arteries affecting a large part of the heart can result in sudden death.

Since the 1950s, doctors have been able to examine the arterial circulation of the heart using angiography. The procedure involves the insertion of a thin flexible tube, or catheter, into an artery.

A radiologist gently threads the catheter through to the artery that needs studying. Then a dye is injected which looks opaque on an X-ray. Therefore where blood flows easily it will show up opaque, and where it does not, there will be nothing visible.

Using this technology, cardiac surgeons were able to see the exact location of any coronary blockage. The next step was to restore the blood flow using a bypass graft technique.

René Gerónimo Favaloro, an Argentinian, was the first to develop this technique while working in the Department of Thoracic and Cardiovascular Surgery in Cleveland, Ohio. Using a vein graft taken from the leg, Favaloro proposed using it to create a detour or 'bypass' around the blockage to restore the blood supply to the heart muscle. The vein he chose was called the saphenous vein. There are other veins in the legs that can do the same job as this one, and so it can be removed without harming the patient.

The first patient to benefit from the technique of Coronary–Artery Bypass Grafting using a vein graft was a 51-year-old woman, and the operation took place on 9 May 1967.

With the advances in interventional radiology, it is now possible to dilate blocked arteries using angioplasty and by inserting stents which are made of wire mesh and designed to hold each artery open.

See: *Angioplasty,* pages 157–158; *Coronary Arterial Stents*, pages 191–192

Palliative Care and the Hospice Movement

Dame Cicely Saunders (1918–2005)

Before Dame Cicely Saunders opened the first modern hospice, the terminally ill had been cared for in hospices mostly run by nuns, where there was little or no medical knowledge or relief from painful or troublesome symptoms.

By the 19th century, medicine had advanced and hospitals were no longer appropriate places for incurable patients who might be seen as medical 'failures'. Gradually, it became clear that dying patients needed a different kind of care.

In France, Jeanne Garnier, a widow and bereaved mother, formed L'Association des Dames de Calaire, in Lyon in 1842 in response to this need. Her idea was to provide sanctuary for the dying. Other similar institutions followed in Paris and New York.

Later, the Irish Sisters of Charity opened Our Lady's Hospice in Dublin in 1879, following this with similar hospices in Australia, Scotland and England. In 1893, the Home for the Dying Poor was opened at St Luke's Hospital in London, followed in 1905 by St Joseph's Hospice in Hackney, London.

Although all of these places provided a shared belief in the importance of providing care for the dying, none were providing medical expertise or further research into the subject.

In the 1960s there was a shift in the way the medical profession began to view the process of dying. Doctors began to take a more positive attitude to terminally ill patients and there was a growing interest in the field of palliative medicine designed to relieve symptoms rather than cure them.

Inspired by her experience as a nurse at St Lukes and St Joseph's, Cicely Saunders served as a medical social worker before deciding to train as a doctor. She graduated from St Thomas' Medical School, London, in 1957, and in 1967 she founded St Christopher's Hospice. Saunders believed that dying was a part of living and didn't need to be a painful, bleak experience. St Christopher's was the first modern hospice where their work was based on the principles of excellent medical care, education for nurses and doctors and research into terminal disease treatments. It also was one of the first hospitals to include the ideas of spiritual as well as medical treatment. This combination of physical and spiritual care alongside scientific research brought about a new approach to the care of the terminally ill and created a change in attitude within the medical profession as a whole.

Dame Cicely Saunders died of cancer at St Christopher's Hospice, aged 87.

First Heart Transplant

Christiaan Barnard (1922–2001)

Successfully transplanting the human heart marked a huge technological breakthrough in the history of medicine.

B arnard's interest in heart transplants began when he saw a patient have a baby with a heart disorder. The condition was untreatable and the child died.

After beginning his career as a general practitioner, he studied transplant surgery in the United States, returning to Cape Town to set up a cardiac unit. After successfully learning to transplant kidneys, his attention turned to hearts.

The ability to transplant the heart relied on the earlier invention of the heart–lung machine. Using this technology, the first successful transplant was carried out in 1967, from 25-year-old road accident victim Denise Darvall into the body of 59-year-old dentist Louis Washkansky, in Cape Town's Groote Schuur Hospital in a nine-hour operation.

In order to help reduce the chance of the transplanting organ being rejected, Washkansky was given large doses of powerful medication. However, sadly this meant that when he caught pneumonia, the very drugs that were supporting his heart, prevented him from fighting the infection and he died 18 days after the transplant.

When asked what was his biggest achievement in life, Barnard replied:

'It's difficult to say. If you ask me what I would like to be remembered for, I would not say the transplants but the surgery I have performed on children with abnormal hearts. It is much more difficult than transplantation and much more satisfying. With the surgical facilities we give a child a chance to lead a normal life.'

The Abortion Act

Before the Abortion Act was passed in the United Kingdom in 1967, around 40 women a year died from back-street abortions.

Even in the 21st century the Abortion Act remains controversial. Although most people in the United Kingdom support the provision of legal abortion, there is still fierce debate surrounding the issue, with several pro-life groups actively campaigning to reduce or remove its availability.

In the Middle Ages, abortion was considered acceptable practice until the woman was around 16–20 weeks pregnant. This was usually when the baby's movements could be felt for the first time, and was when the soul first entered the foetus, according to the Church. This view remained unchanged for centuries, and was reinforced by the Ellenborough Act in 1803 when it became illegal to carry out an abortion after the movements could be felt, and the punishment for breaking the law was the death penalty.

In 1837 the Act was amended so that abortion became illegal altogether. But these laws didn't stop the need for abortion, and thousands of women resorted to back-street abortionists. Many women died or became permanently infertile as a result.

Concerns about the risks to women's health led to campaign groups calling for reforms to the law. In 1929 it became legal to perform an abortion in exceptional cases, when the mother's life was at risk. This was known as the Infant Life Preservation Act.

The next major change came in 1938. In a landmark case, Dr Alex Bourne was acquitted of having performed an illegal abortion on a 14-year-old girl who had been raped. This set a precedent for future doctors to carry out similar abortions when the woman's future mental health (as well as her physical health) was considered to be at risk.

Nearly 30 years later the Abortion Act of 1967 came into force legalizing abortion under certain conditions. In 1990, the law was amended by the Human Fertilisation and Embryology Act to lower the legal time limit to below 24 weeks. The Act allowed abortion with the signature of two doctors, on condition that one or more of the following was satisfied:

1. the pregnancy was less than 24 weeks and continuing the pregnancy would involve a greater risk to the physical or mental health of a pregnant woman or her family than if the baby was born.

2. there was a risk that the child would be born physically or mentally disabled.
3. the abortion was necessary to prevent grave permanent injury to the mental or physical health of the woman.
4. continuing the pregnancy would involve risk to the life of the pregnant woman, greater than if the pregnancy were terminated.

The Act also stated that In the event of an abortion being needed as a matter of medical emergency a second doctor's agreement need not be sought.

Folic Acid and the Link with Neural Tube Defects

Richard Smithells (1924–2002)

Neural tube defects are disorders of the developing spine, spinal cord or brain in a foetus.

The most common neural tube defect is spina bifida, which occurs when some of the developing spinal cord bulges out through an opening in the spine.

The successful identification of folic acid deficiency as a major contributor to the development of a neural tube defect in pregnancy led to the introduction of advice to all women to take folic acid supplements before and during early pregnancy. This action has dramatically reduced the numbers of affected children.

Neural tube defects were known to be more common in women from poorer households, and the link with their diet had already been established. However, it was Richard Smithells, a Liverpool paediatrician, who was the first to suggest that it might be to do with the mother's intake of folic acid.

The spinal cord and brain are fully developed just one month after conception, at a stage when many women do not yet know they are pregnant. Smithell's team showed that giving women a vitamin containing 360 micrograms of folic acid several weeks before conception and during the early weeks of pregnancy was linked with a lower rate of neural tube defects in their children. His research was published in 1968 and prompted a bigger and better trial run by the Medical Research Council (MRC) in 1983 to confirm his results.

The MRC's randomized double blind controlled trial in 33 centres looked at whether folic acid supplements or a mixture of seven other vitamins (A, D,

B1, B4, B6, C and nicotinamide) around the time of conception could reduce the chance of having a baby with a neural tube defect. The results showed that women taking folic acid were 72 per cent less likely to have an affected child. There was no change in the risk for women taking the other vitamins.

Within weeks the US Centres for Disease Control (CDC) had issued guidance to all women to encourage them to increase the amount of folic acid in their diet from foods like brussel sprouts, green beans, oranges, yeast and beef extracts. For women with a higher risk of having a baby with neural tube defects, that is, those who already had an affected child, the CDC recommended taking supplements around the time of conception.

A year later, the CDC recommended that all women planning a pregnancy should take 400 micrograms of folic acid every day before pregnancy and for the first three months because it is unlikely that they can get the sufficient amount from diet alone. Women with a previous child affected by neural tube defects were advised to take a higher dose of 5mg daily for the same time period. Other countries followed suit with similar advice soon afterwards.

See: *Randomized–Controlled Trials,* page 121

Salbutamol

David Jack (b. 1924)

During an asthma attack the muscle in the airways tightens, making it harder to breathe in and out – a bit like trying to breathe through a straw. Salbutamol works by relaxing the muscle, the equivalent of making the straw much bigger, and therefore air can flow more easily.

David Jack was the sixth son of a coal miner in Fife. Breaking from tradition, he became an apprentice pharmacist at Boots the chemist, and later joined the drug company Glaxo as a researcher. He eventually became Director of Research and Development and is credited with the discovery of Salbutamol.

Jack's findings were based on the discovery in 1903 that adrenaline could relieve asthma, but it also had unwanted effects on the cardiovascular system – in particular causing a rapid rise in blood pressure. In the late 1940s, different types of adrenaline receptor were discovered. These receptors, or adrenoreceptors as they are known, are areas of the cell membrane that the adrenaline stimulates to produce its effect. As it later turned out, there are actually two types of adrenoreceptor – type one and type two – discovered in 1967. Type one receptors are mainly in the heart, and type two are in the muscles of the airway.

Jack discovered that salbutamol stimulates only type two receptors, relieving symptoms in asthma, whereas adrenaline stimulates both types. In addition, Salbutamol acts quickly, giving almost instant relief from asthma attacks, and lasts up to six hours.

Subsequent developments led to the introduction in the 1990s of a longer acting version – lasting twelve hours or more, so that medication only needs to be taken once or twice a day.

The Five Stages of Grief

Elisabeth Kübler-Ross (1926–2004)

Before Elisabeth Kübler-Ross published her book, On Death and Dying, *in 1969, death was taboo and dying patients were an embarrassing admission of failure for most doctors.*

Before the late 1960s, dying patients were ignored on hospital wards and medical students were not taught about death and bereavement.

Elisabeth Kübler Ross, an American psychiatrist originally from Switzerland, disagreed with this attitude towards the dying. She was strongly influenced in her work by Dame Cicely Saunders (1918–2005), founder of the modern hospice movement. Saunders believed that dying patients could be treated with dignity and enabled to die with minimal discomfort.

Kübler-Ross began to give lectures to medical students on death and dying, forcing them to confront the issue. She also interviewed dying patients and wrote a book based on her findings, describing 'five stages of grief' – denial, anger, bargaining, depression and acceptance (*see illustration opposite*). According to her now widely accepted view, patients and their families experience these stages in the months and years after a terminal diagnosis.

In the first stage, denial, there is a refusal to accept the facts. Stage two, anger, can be directed inwards or outwards towards others. After anger comes bargaining. Traditionally this can involve religion, calling on God to help solve the crisis. Depression, stage four, is sometimes thought to be a preparation for death and grieving and precedes a stage of calm acceptance.

Kübler-Ross believed that the stages of grief could happen in any order, and might not be completed, but they were recognizable in most people.

The book and its ideas were quite revolutionary at the time, and were a catalyst for a change in the way doctors and nurses understood and cared for dying patients and their families.

See: *Palliative Care and the Hospice Movement*, pages 162–163

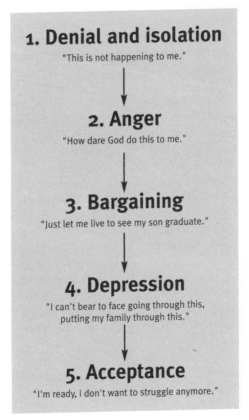

1. Denial and isolation
"This is not happening to me."

2. Anger
"How dare God do this to me."

3. Bargaining
"Just let me live to see my son graduate."

4. Depression
"I can't bear to face going through this, putting my family through this."

5. Acceptance
"I'm ready, I don't want to struggle anymore."

Tamoxifen for Breast Cancer

Arthur L. Walpole (d. 1977)

In the past 25 years the number of new cases of breast cancer has increased dramatically, and worldwide more than a million women are now diagnosed with breast cancer every year.

The highest rates of breast cancer are in Northern Europe and North America, while parts of Africa and Asia have the world's lowest rates. In the United Kingdom it is now the most common cancer with 44,000 newly diagnosed women every year – that is more than 100 every day. The drug Tamoxifen has been one of the biggest breakthroughs in the treatment of the disease.

When tamoxifen came on the scene in the 1970s, the standard treatment for breast cancer was to remove the whole breast in a disfiguring operation, possibly followed by radiotherapy. Recurrent cancer was common, and less than half of sufferers survived more than 10 years after the diagnosis. But by the

1990s, following the widespread introduction of tamoxifen, women with breast cancer were surviving long enough to die from other causes.

Tamoxifen was discovered in the late 1950s in the research laboratories of ICI Pharmaceuticals (now AstraZeneca). Arthur Walpole, a doctor interested in the hormones of reproduction, was leading a team that was investigating tamoxifen as a possible morning-after contraceptive pill because it was known to block the effects of oestrogen. Unfortunately tamoxifen seemed to have the opposite effect – actually promoting ovulation – so it was abandoned for this purpose. For a while, there seemed to be no disease that could benefit from tamoxifen's effects.

At around the same time, researchers

Tamoxifen.

elsewhere were studying why it was that some women with breast cancer improved after their ovaries were removed and others did not. Eventually, they realized that some breast cancer cells have proteins called receptors on their surface to which oestrogen attaches, triggering the growth and division of the cancer cell. Only some cancers have the oestrogen receptors, and it is these that respond to the removal of the ovaries, and therefore the reduction in the circulating oestrogen.

Realizing that tamoxifen might be helpful in blocking breast cancer oestrogen receptor cells, Walpole supported the ongoing research, although ICI was less interested because breast cancer was not a priority at the time. He passed on his ideas to doctors working at the nearby Christie Hospital in Manchester, and encouraged them to start a clinical trial on the use of the drug in women with cancer. He also supported the work of a little-known pharmacologist called Craig Jordan, who was working on oestrogen receptors. At one stage he was sending Jordan 200 rats a week in a chauffeur-driven car for use in his experiments!

After more research, Walpole's efforts were finally rewarded, as the medical community was convinced by the findings that women with oestrogen receptor positive breast cancer responded very positively to treatment with tamoxifen. ICI finally marketed tamoxifen as a treatment for breast cancer in 1973. By May 2000 up to 20,000 lives had been saved.

Although there have been improvements in early diagnosis and surgery that have also contributed to this figure, experts estimate that two thirds of these women were saved by tamoxifen.

Pregnancy Tests

It seems extraordinary now to think that when the contraceptive pill was introduced in 1960, we still didn't have an easy way of diagnosing a pregnancy.

These days, pregnancy-testing kits are available over the counter and can diagnose a pregnancy in a couple of minutes, but it wasn't always this easy.

Doctors have known for thousands of years that there is something different about the urine of a pregnant woman. According to one ancient Egyptian papyrus, if a woman urinated on wheat or barley seeds, they would grow if she was pregnant. However, until the development of a more reliable pregnancy test than this, doctors and women had to rely on physical symptoms and signs to diagnose a pregnancy.

Women often thought they might be pregnant if their periods stopped and they were experiencing morning sickness and breast tenderness. Their doctors relied on signs such as Chadwick's signs, discovered by the French physician Etienne Joseph Jacquemin (1796–1872), who described a bluish discoloration of the vaginal tissue, vulva and cervix due to extra blood flowing through the veins in the area, visible 6–8 weeks following conception.

Doctors also used Hegar's sign, first described by German physician Ernst Ludwig Alfred Hegar(1830–1914) in 1895. In this sign, the examining doctor can feel softening in the lower part of the womb (just above the cervix but below the very top of the uterus) in the first part of the pregnancy.

Of course, a pregnancy could be diagnosed by a foetal heartbeat by listening with a Pinard stethoscope, but this was only possible from around 20 weeks onwards.

By the beginning of the 20th century, researchers had identified some of the hormones important in reproduction. However, it wasn't until 1970 that the first pregnancy testing kit became available.

Isotretinoin for Acne

Acne affects most teenagers at some stage, but isn't exclusive to this age group. It often occurs in adults in their 30s and even 40s.

This embarrassing skin condition causes discomfort and can lead to feelings of low self-esteem and depression. Prior to the introduction of Isotretinoin, the only treatment available for severe acne was long-term treatment with antibiotics.

Isotretinoin is known as Accutane® in the United States and Roaccutane® in Britain. It is a derivative of Vitamin A, which is known to be important in maintaining normal reproduction, vision and healthy looking skin. However, Vitamin A has side effects which have limited its use as a treatment.

In the 1950s researchers discovered Vitamin A derivatives – retinoids – that were less toxic than Vitamin A and could be used to treat acne. This was a significant discovery previously as the main treatment of moderate to severe or persistent acne was over-the-counter benzoyl peroxide (which dries out the skin) usually combined with antibiotic lotions or antibiotic tablets. Although the antibiotics do work, they tend to become less effective with time as the bacteria contributing to the acne develop resistance to the antibiotics.

Isotretinoin was the first retinoid to be synthesized in 1955, and was formed by modification of the Vitamin A molecule. It was initially used to treat psoriasis and subsequently found to be highly effective in the treatment of severe acne, and acne that hasn't responded to less potent medicines. Initial studies found that 13 out of 14 patients given isotretinoin treatment for four months were completely clear of acne after the treatment, and remained free of spots for five years after the treatment stopped.

Isotretinoin reduces the production of oil (sebum), the size of oil producing glands and prevents blackheads forming.

Computerized Tomography (CT)

Godfrey Hounsfield (1919–2004)
Alan Cormack (1924–1998)

When a computer combines many x-rays of the same area to create a cross-sectional image, the result is called a CT scan. Cormack and Hounsfield worked independently.

In 1979, Alan Cormack and Godfrey Hounsfield were awarded the Nobel Prize for medicine for their groundbreaking research.

Cormack was a South African-born physicist. In 1957 he moved to the United States, where he worked mainly on particle physics while also developing his interest in X-rays. He published two papers summarizing the theoretical concepts of computerized tomography in the *Journal of Applied Physics* in 1963 and 1964.

Hounsfield was an engineer working at EMI Laboratories in Middlesex, England, where he worked for a while on radar and guided weapons. He was among the first to work on the development of computers in the 1950s.

In the 1960s he became interested in the idea of computerized tomography. In some of Hounsfield's initial experiments using the early machines, he used the organs from dead animals. In one instance he described travelling across London on public transport with a bullock's brain in his bag.

The first CT scanners for patient use were installed in 1975, and initially were just used for scanning the head. Whole body CT scanners became available a year later.

Since the initial machines, there have been many modifications and modern CT scanners are faster and more detailed than their predecessors.

Evidence-based Medicine

Archie Cochrane (1908–1988)

*Evidence-based medicine is not supposed to
replace individual clinical expertise and experience,
but rather to inform it and be integrated
into clinical decision-making.*

Before the advent of evidence-based medicine, a doctor's authority was considered to be sufficient evidence and wasn't questioned. Doctors didn't need research evidence to support their authority: they based their advice on clinical experience and medical knowledge. This model for clinical practice has now been largely replaced by a system whereby clinicians share the best available research evidence with their patients. Suitable treatment options are then formulated for each individual patient.

The concept developed from the randomized-controlled trial research methodology, popularized in the late 1940s, and has become one of the driving forces in 21st century medicine, impacting on education, policy-making, and research.

The most significant driver behind the concept of evidence based medicine was Archie Cochrane, a Scottish epidemiologist, through his influential book, *Effectiveness and Efficiency: Random Reflections on Health Services*, published in 1972, although the term 'evidence-based medicine' wasn't actually coined until the 1990s.

In his book, Cochrane argued that as resources would always be limited, they should be allocated according to what was proven to be most effective, and that the evidence for this should come from randomized-controlled trials.

Evidence-based medicine also relies on good systems for disseminating the knowledge to clinicians in practice.

Cholesterol-lowering Drugs

Akira Endo (b.1933)

*Cholesterol-lowering drugs, or statins as they
are more often known, are responsible for
lowering blood cholesterol levels and reducing
the risk of heart disease and strokes.*

Akira Endo, a Japanese biochemist first discovered statins via his interest in moulds. After his initial training Endo joined Sankyo, a pharmaceutical company based in Tokyo, where his job was to research food ingredients and find an enzyme to make fruit juice less pulpy. Sankyo rewarded his success with a trip to the New York Albert Einstein College of Medicine in 1966 to pursue his research in cholesterol – a popular subject for ambitious scientists at the time.

Although cholesterol intake is an important factor in the cholesterol level in the body, the liver makes most of the body's cholesterol. Like all fats, cholesterol is not soluble in water, so it is transported around the blood stream attached to a protein, as lipoprotein.

There are different types: low-density lipoprotein (LDL) and very low-density lipoprotein (VLDL), which carry cholesterol to the tissues. High levels of VLDL and LDL are linked with heart disease. High-density lipoprotein, (HDL), carries cholesterol back to the liver. Lots of HDL therefore protects against cardiovascular disease. Blocking the production of cholesterol in the liver also stimulates the clearance of LDL from the bloodstream and therefore a decrease in blood cholesterol levels.

When Endo was researching cholesterol, a lot was already known about it in the body. Several researchers had already shown that blocking an enzyme called HMG-CoA reductase might provide a way for manufacturing a drug to reduce cholesterol levels.

Endo thought that fungi probably employed chemicals to protect themselves from parasitic bacteria by preventing the synthesis of cholesterol, an essential ingredient in the manufacture of cell walls, without which the parasite could not survive. He thought that if he could identify these chemicals it might prove useful in preventing cholesterol synthesis in people with raised cholesterol levels.

He went back to Tokyo and persuaded Sankyo to give him funding to pursue his theory. In 1971 Endo and another chemist, Masao Kuroda, along with two laboratory assistants started their search. They studied 6,000 moulds. Each one was tested for its ability to block HMG-CoA reductase. After two years they eventually found three from the fungus *Penicillium citrinum*. One of these, mevastatin, became the first statin.

Endo's initial success met with disinterest. Convinced that he was onto something, he persuaded Akira Yamamoto a physician at Osaka University hospital to try out his new drugs in patients with inherited high cholesterol levels. There was no ethics committee and some patients experienced unpleasant muscle pains. However, their cholesterol levels fell, and when Sankyo saw the results, it agreed to test Endo's drug further.

In 1976, the pharmaceutical company Merck & Co. began to show an interest in Japan's research into statins after Sankyo allowed them access to Endo's files. In 1978 it isolated another similar chemical that it called lovastatin, from the mould Aspergillus terreus. This became the first commercially marketed statin although it didn't get approval from the US Food and Drug Administration until 1987. (Unfortunately Endo didn't benefit financially because Sankyo failed to negotiate a fee for him should Merck find the drug before Endo did.)

Evidence of the value of statins followed, with numerous research trials showing that taking statins can reduce the risk of heart disease and stroke in people who have already got heart disease or had a stroke. Treatment is also recommended for people with no history of disease but who have a high overall risk – such as diabetics and heavy smokers.

In 2004, Endo's doctors found he had raised LDL cholesterol. Surprisingly, Endo didn't take the statins as he was advised by his doctor, quoting the Japanese proverb as his reason: *The indigo dyer wears white trousers.*

Positron Emission Tomography (PET Scans)

Michael E. Phelps (b. 1939)

The invention of PET Scans enabled doctors to look at how different parts of the body function, and to identify cancers at an early stage of development.

Before the invention of PET, scan-imaging techniques, such as CT and MRI scans, were only able to show the anatomical structure of the body.

Michael Phelps invented the technique while working as a biophysicist at Washington University School of Medicine. His design used low doses of radioactive sugar injected into a vein to measure the activity and function of different organs in the body.

Because cancers use glucose faster than normal areas, they look more prominent on a PET scan, which makes it possible to diagnose early cancers and monitor their progress through a course of treatment.

PET scans are also useful to show how different parts of the brain work, which can be helpful after a stroke or in the study of brain diseases such as dementia and Parkinson's disease.

The most commonly used radioactive drug is fluorine 18, also known as FDG-18, a radioactive version of glucose. But despite the use of radiation, the technique is considered to be very safe with the exposure to radiation being similar to having an X-ray.

The scan involves lying on a couch, which moves through a large ring-shaped scanner containing sensors. These detect the gamma ray signals given off by the radioactive material. A computer then reassembles the signals and turns them into images. Depending on the area that is being scanned, the examination (and the preparation time) can last up to two hours.

The early PET scans were complex to perform and needed a large staff including physicists, chemists and physicians. But during the 1980s the technology underlying PET advanced greatly. Commercial PET scanners were developed with more precise resolution and images. As a result, many of the steps required for producing a PET scan became automated and could be performed by a trained technician and experienced physician, thereby reducing the cost and complexity of the procedure.

Cochlear Implants

Adam Kissiah (b.1929)

A small electronic device implanted behind the ear can restore hearing to profoundly deaf children and adults.

The experiments that led to the development of the cochlear implant began in 1950s California. However it was not until 1977 that the real breakthrough came.

Adam Kissiah, a NASA engineer with no medical background, became interested in the field of acoustics when he began to lose his own hearing. Using his knowledge of electronics, he designed a cochlear implant that was so successful that it is still widely used today.

The device consists of a microphone and a sound processor. The processor selects and arranges sounds that are detected by the microphone. There is also a transmitter and a receiver. The receiver converts signals from the speech processor into electrical impulses. Lastly, a group of electrodes collect information from the receiver and send them to different parts of the auditory nerve.

Although the device doesn't restore normal hearing, it can help a deaf person to hear sounds and understand speech.

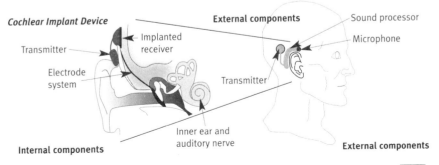

Cochlear Implant Device

External components — Sound processor

Transmitter — Implanted receiver — Microphone

Electrode system — Transmitter

Internal components — Inner ear and auditory nerve — External components

Magnetic Resonance Imaging (MRI)

Raymond Damadian (b. 1936)

Magnetic resonance imaging produces detailed three-dimensional images of the body without the need for surgery, harmful dyes or radiation.

———

The MRI method uses a technique originally called Nuclear Magnetic Resonance Imaging (the word nuclear was later dropped), based on the concept of nuclear magnetic resonance, which was discovered originally in the 1930s. In 1952 Felix Bloch (1905–1983) and Edward Purcell (b.1912) were awarded the Nobel Prize for Physics for their work in this area.

In principle, what Bloch and Purcell discovered was that when hydrogen atoms are bombarded with energy from magnets, they resonate, giving off radio waves. Given that the human body is primarily made of fat and water, it contains a lot of hydrogen atoms capable of resonating in this way.

In the 1970s Raymond Damadian found that various kinds of animal tissue emit response signals of differing length. He also discovered a diversity in response signals between cancerous and non-cancerous tissue, and among response times of other kinds of diseased tissue.

Damadian and his team completed the first MRI scanner in 1977, which he called *Indomitable* because it had taken seven years to complete it. The machine was a hollow cylinder containing a strong electromagnet to produce a magnetic field.

Damadian's assistant Larry Minkoff was the first to try the machine because Damadian wasn't slim enough. Damadian obtained a patent for his design in 1974 and established the FONAR Corporation in 1978, which introduced the first commercial MRI scanner in 1980.

MRI Scanner Cutaway

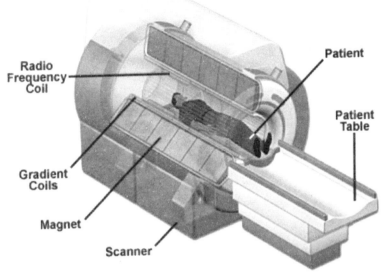

An MRI scanner.

In-Vitro Fertilization (IVF)

Patrick Steptoe (1913–1988)
Robert Edwards (b.1925)

When it was introduced, IVF was hailed as a great success in the treatment of infertile couples.

There has been a rapid expansion of research into infertility since the discovery of IVF and much debate about the ethics of treating infertile couples.

Patrick Steptoe and Robert Edwards originally worked separately before combining their knowledge to develop IVF. Edwards, a physiologist in Cambridge, was studying human fertilization in his laboratory using eggs from ovaries that had been removed surgically. He developed a chemically balanced fluid that kept the eggs alive in the laboratory, and in 1968 successfully fertilised one of the eggs. Describing the moment years later Edwards said: *'It was amazing. Then, I knew that the whole field was opening up before my eyes.'*

Edwards' work was based on the foundations laid originally by another British physiologist: Walter Heape (1855–1929) who, in 1890, had been the first to remove an embryo from the fallopian tube of a rabbit and transfer it to a foster mother rabbit, resulting in a normal pregnancy. His work encouraged others to further research the possibility of growing embryos in the laboratory.

At the same time as Edwards, Patrick Steptoe, a gynaecologist in Oldham, Greater Manchester was working with the newly introduced keyhole-surgery techniques. Recognizing the potential for collaboration, the two men met in 1968 and began combined research.

Using eggs collected from the ovaries of healthy volunteers the two men perfected the best time to collect the eggs, and the ideal conditions for fertilization in the laboratory.

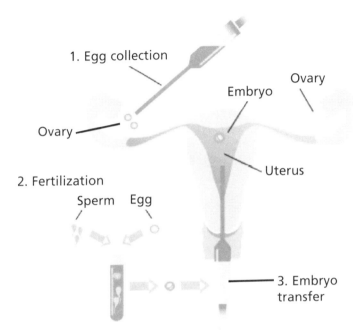

1. Egg collection

Embryo

Ovary

Ovary

2. Fertilization

Sperm   Egg

Uterus

3. Embryo transfer

The process of in-vitro fertilization.

Their work was helped by the expansion in knowledge about human hormones, and their role in controlling reproduction. In order to maximize the chances of successful IVF, the woman is given hormones for about two weeks prior to egg collection, and intensively monitored with blood tests and ultrasound to determine the optimum time to collect the eggs.

Just before the eggs are due to be released from the ovary they are collected using a hollow needle pushed through the wall of the vagina using local anaesthetic. The eggs are kept in the laboratory in a nutrient mixture, which acts as a substitute for the environment that would otherwise have been provided by the fallopian tubes in a naturally occurring pregnancy.

Once sperm are added, and one or more eggs have fertilized, usually the eggs will develop and the cells will divide a few times to become what's known as 'pre-implantation embryos.'

These are reintroduced into the uterus via the vagina two days after the egg collection and then the wait is on for a successful outcome.

Edwards and Steptoe had their first success in 1975, when a human embryo was successfully replaced into the mother. However, the pregnancy developed in a Fallopian tube, which is known as an ectopic pregnancy, resulting in a miscarriage.

This was followed in 1977 by another successful attempt. A healthy girl, Louise Brown, was born in July 1978, becoming the world's first 'test-tube' baby.

IVF has always been controversial. Church leaders have questioned the ethics of changing the natural course of couple's ability to have children. Others claimed the treatment gives false hope, since the chances of a successful pregnancy are still quite low.

There have also been occasional disasters when the wrong embryo has been re-implanted, adding to the debate about the technique. And then there is the cost – at thousands of pounds for each attempt at pregnancy, and variable state provision for treatment, it remains an option that only some couples can realistically consider.

See: *Keyhole Surgery*, pages 194–195

Botox

Alan B. Scott
Edward J. Schantz (1909–2005)

Introduced originally as a non-surgical treatment for patients with crossed eyes, Botox is now a popular method for reducing the appearance of wrinkles.

Botulinum toxin is a protein produced by the bacteria *Clostridium botulinum* found commonly in soil. It is one of the most poisonous naturally occurring substances, and outbreaks of botulism, although rare, tend to be linked with inadequately processed canned food. The poison works by causing generalised muscle paralysis so the victim dies from suffocation as the breathing muscles stop working.

One of the earliest-documented outbreaks of botulism food poisoning was in Württemberg in south-western Germany in the 18th century. The Württemberg district medical officer - Justinus Kerner (1786–1862), who was also a well-known German poet, was the first to describe the symptoms accurately, and correctly attributed it to a food-borne poison:

> The nerve conduction is brought by the toxin into a condition in which its influence on the chemical process of life is interrupted.

The bacteria *Clostridium botulinum* was eventually discovered in 1895 by Emile Pierre van Ermengem (1851–1932), professor of bacteriology at the University of Ghent, following an outbreak of botulism in all the guests at a funeral party in Ellezelles, a small village in Belgium. All those who ate the smoked ham at the meal became ill. The name '*botulism*' originates from the Latin word '*botulus*', which means sausage.

In the Second World War (1939–1945), the American military turned its attention to Botulinum toxin as a potential biological weapon. Allegedly, the US Office of Strategic Services had a plan to assassinate high-ranking Japanese officers using small gelatin capsules containing a lethal dose of botulinum. Edward Schantz, a biochemist who later became director of food microbiology and toxicology at the University of Wisconsin, worked on the production and evaluation of the poison. He concluded that botulinum had only limited battlefield applications. However, as a result of his work in extracting and purifying the toxin, Schantz was able to supply it to Alan Scott in the 1960s, who at the time was working as a researcher at the Smith–Kettlewell Eye Research Institute in San Francisco in California.

Scott began testing samples of botulinum toxin on monkeys in his search to find a nonsurgical cure for crossed eyes, otherwise known as strabismus. He found that a tiny quantity injected into a specific muscle could paralyse the muscle without having an effect elsewhere on the body.

His work with monkeys was so successful that in 1980 he began using the toxin to treat human patients with strabismus. News of the treatment spread and soon it became an accepted treatment for this condition.

Then there was an unexpected breakthrough. In Vancouver, the ophthalmologist Jean Carruthers noticed that when she treated patients, in addition to reducing the muscle spasm as expected, they also lost the appearance of wrinkles around their eyes. Fortuitously she was married to a dermatologist – Alastair Carruthers – who began using the drug to treat his patients as an alternative to cosmetic surgery. This treatment has been hugely successful, partly because it is a relatively painless, low-cost alternative to cosmetic surgery with minimal side effects.

The drug is now licensed for the treatment of muscle spasms and for the treatment of wrinkles. It is also used to treat excessive sweating in the armpits.

Coronary Arterial Stents

Charles Dotter (1920–1985)

*A stent is a mesh made of wire that keeps
an artery open, like a scaffold.*

Stents are now used widely in the treatment of coronary artery disease, where the blood vessels supplying essential nutrients and oxygen to the heart muscle have become narrowed or blocked.

Since German cardiologist Andreas Gruentzig(1939–1985) invented balloon angioplasty in 1975, cardiologists had been able to insert a small tube, or catheter, into the blocked coronary arteries. When in the correct position, the catheter could be opened wider by inflating a tiny balloon. Sometimes, the wall of the coronary artery was weakened during the process, and occasionally the artery would collapse closed again after the catheter and balloon had been removed. If this happened immediately, the patient might need emergency Coronary-Artery Bypass Grafts.

The narrowing could also happen slowly, and around a third of all arteries treated would close up gradually. Radiologists and cardiologists began to look for a solution.

The solution was the stent first invented in 1969 by Charles Dotter, a radiologist in Oregon, when he successfully implanted one in a dog. After years of refining his design, in 1983, he and colleague Andrew Craig came up with an expandable tubular shaped stent made out of nitinol, an elastic alloy that remembers its original shape even when it has been stretched for a long period. When collapsed, the stent can be inserted into an artery. When it's in position, it expands to its original shape, holding the artery open, and thereby helping to improve blood flow.

Dotter, who is widely credited as the founder of interventional radiology, said of his work: *'It's a gross oversimplification, of course, but ... if a plumber can do it to pipes, we can do it to blood vessels.'*

Stents stopped the problem of sudden artery closure, but at around six months after the procedure around a quarter still closed up. The next development was drug-eluting stents. These are normal stents coated in a medicine that's known to prevent the process of blocking closed. This has reduced the number of stents that block to single figures.

See: *Coronary–Artery Bypass Grafting*, pages 160–161;
Angioplasty, pages 157–158

Egg Donation

Peter Lutjen, Alan Trounson and colleagues

Pregnancy using donated eggs is the only option for women who have had an early menopause (either naturally or through cancer treatment) or who have left it too late to conceive naturally. It is also used to help women who carry a genetic defect and cannot conceive a foetus using their own eggs without passing on the disorder.

Although the first significant breakthrough in infertility treatment was in the United Kingdom with the first birth from in-vitro fertilization (IVF) in 1978, most of the following developments, including egg donation, took place in Australia.

Gynaecologist Peter Lutjen and biologist Alan Trounson together with a team of scientists at the Queen Victoria Medical Centre (now part of the Monash Medical Centre) in Melbourne, became the first to achieve a pregnancy and birth in an infertile woman using her husband's sperm and donated eggs.

In the procedure, eggs are collected from the donor, and then fertilized using IVF. The fertilized eggs are reimplanted into the infertile woman. This enables her to achieve a pregnancy using her partner's sperm, although not her own egg.

The success rate of IVF using donor eggs can be high – often more than 50 per cent – and the younger the age of the donor, the higher the success rate of the IVF.

Waiting lists for egg donation vary, but are lower in countries such as the United States, where donors often receive money.

See: *In-Vitro Fertilization (IVF)*, pages 186–188

Keyhole Surgery

Kurt Semm (1927–2003)

*Until the invention of keyhole surgery,
having an operation usually meant a big scar and
several days, at least, in hospital. Now surgeons
can learn to operate through a much smaller cut,
perhaps only a few centimetres. With this discovery,
patients experience far less pain, minimal scarring
and have a shorter stay in hospital.*

For more than two thousand years, doctors have been using instruments to look inside the body's cavities. The procedure, known as endoscopy, makes use of existing bodily orifices like the mouth, or anus or vagina, to gain access to the inside of the body.

It was not until the 19th century that doctors began to exploit this technique further. First they began to use tubular endoscopes, with a system of lights and mirrors to get a better view inside the body. The earliest light sources were naked flames, which occasionally ran the risk of burning the patient. By the end of the 19th century, endoscopes contained miniature electric lights.

At the turn of the 20th century, surgeons began to experiment by making holes in the chest and abdomen to examine the interior of the body. Using an endoscope to examine the abdominal cavity became known as a laparoscopy.

By the 1930s, the invention of fibre-optics meant the light source could be incorporated into a flexible and thinner endoscope. And at the same time, new instruments were designed that could be passed into the body cavity via small incisions, such as forceps, and miniature lasers. In the 1970s it became possible to attach miniature cameras to endoscopes allowing surgeons to look at images on a screen of the inside of the body.

These developments allowed surgeons to consider the possibility of operating via endoscopy. Kurt Semm was a gynaecologist at the University of Kiel in Germany and had been experimenting with the use of laparoscopy for surgery for some years despite opposition from his colleagues. At the time, it was considered dangerous to operate without being able to see and feel the organs that were being removed. His techniques were considered so dangerous that after his appointment as Professor of Obstetrics and Gynaecology Semm's colleagues insisted that he have a brain scan because they thought he might be suffering from brain damage!

However, despite derision from contemporaries, in 1980 Semm performed an appendectomy, the world's first surgical procedure via laparoscope.

His work caught the attention of European surgeons and in 1985 Erich Mühe at the University of Böblingen did the first laparoscopic cholecystecomy, (gall bladder removal). Soon more surgeons were trying the technique and just a few years later, in 1990, the European Association of Endoscopic Surgery (EAES) was founded in Paris. Within two years, most surgeons in Europe were operating using minimally invasive techniques.

Preimplantation Genetic Diagnosis

Alan Handyside
Robert Winston (b.1940)

Whereas previously it was only possible to diagnose some genetic disorders in pregnancy using ultrasound and amniocentesis, with preimplantation diagnosis, a genetic disorder can be detected in the laboratory when the embryo is only a clump of cells in a Petri dish.

Preimplantation genetic diagnosis was pioneered at the Hammersmith Hospital in London where Alan Handyside and Robert Winston led a team of scientists in their research into cystic fibrosis.

After a woman's eggs were collected during IVF they removed a single cell from a two- or three-day-old embryo. Using highly specialized diagnostic techniques, they found they could search for a single gene in the DNA of the removed cell. The DNA weighed just six-trillionth of a gram.

Handyside and his colleagues used a technique called '*nested primer polymerase chain reaction*' to find the gene. This involves amplifying a piece of DNA, then amplifying the DNA within the amplified segments. Embryos found to carry the gene coding for cystic fibrosis were allowed to die, and only those not coding for the disease were reimplanted into the woman.

Three couples were involved in the groundbreaking research. In all cases both the man and the woman carried one copy of the cystic fibrosis gene. Although the parents were unaffected by the disease, any child who inherited one copy of the cystic fibrosis gene from each parent would have the disease and every time the couple conceived there was a one in four chance of this happening.

The first couple had five embryos. Two embryos each had two copies of the cystic fibrosis gene, two had one copy each of the gene, and the fifth had no copies of the defective gene. The couple chose to have one of the embryos containing one copy of the cystic fibrosis gene implanted, and also the unaffected embryo. However, the woman did not become pregnant.

A second couple had two embryos. The gene analysis was unsuccessful with one of them, and the other embryo had two copies of the cystic fibrosis gene, so none were transferred into the woman.

The third couple had six embryos. Two had two copies of the cystic fibrosis gene, two had no copies of the gene, one had one copy of the gene and in one the genetic analysis was unsuccessful. The couple had two embryos transferred – one with a single copy of the defective gene and one with no copy of the gene. In 1988 the woman gave birth to a baby girl, and as predicted, she did not have cystic fibrosis. Further testing revealed the baby had no copies of the gene.

Preimplantation genetic diagnosis has since developed to enable scientists to detect a limited number of inherited genetic conditions including haemophilia and sickle cell disease. However, the technology has provoked widespread ethical debate about the morals of discarding 'faulty' embryos. Supporters argue that there is a distinction between an embryo in a Petri dish and a foetus in the womb. Discarding embryos is not considered to be the moral equivalent to abortion.

The technique can accurately diagnose the sex of an embryo, which is vital in the diagnosis of inherited conditions that affect one sex only, such as haemophilia. Opponents are worried that the technique could be used to select embryos of one gender in order for a family to have the child of their choice. And as the technology progresses, potentially the condition could be used to select for other characteristics too, such as eye colour, hair colour and so on, the so called 'designer baby'. Strict codes of practice are in place to limit the use and prevent abuse of preimplantation genetic diagnosis.

See: *In-Vitro Fertilization (IVF)*, pages 186–188

Surfactant for Premature Babies

John Allen Clements

Before the discovery of synthetic surfactant as a treatment, many babies born too early died from breathing problems due to their under-developed lungs.

Premature babies dying from breathing problems famously included Patrick Bouvier Kennedy, the infant son of John F. Kennedy, President of the United States (1917–1963; in office 1961–1963) and his wife Jacqueline (1929–1994), who was born nearly six weeks early and who died in August 1963, aged just two days.

Most pregnancies last around 40 weeks. Any baby born before 37 weeks of pregnancy is premature, and is more likely to have health problems.

This is partly because in the last few weeks of pregnancy, the foetus develops a protein in the lungs called surfactant. If the baby is born before surfactant develops, it is likely to have breathing difficulties because surfactant stops the small air sacs in the lungs from collapsing every time the baby breathes out.

John Clements, an American physiologist, first identified surfactant in 1959. Lots of research studies followed, trying to find a way of making surfactant and treating premature babies, with limited success.

In the 1980s Clements was the first to develop a synthetic version of the natural surfactant, which, after a few feasibility studies, rapidly gained approval for widespread use in 1990. (In fact, because of its importance, the drug was widely available in 1989 while it was still experimental.)

Lots of similar synthetic surfactants followed, but this first surfactant was known as Exosurf® and was supplied as a powder, to be dissolved in sterile water and then given through a tube into the windpipe while a machine ventilated the baby.

By 1990, an estimated 30,000 infants in 500 hospitals in North America, Europe and Japan had been enrolled in clinical trials of different surfactant replacements, many of which also gained approval. The treatment has been so successful that since 1990 the number of babies dying from respiratory problems due to their prematurity has been halved as a result.

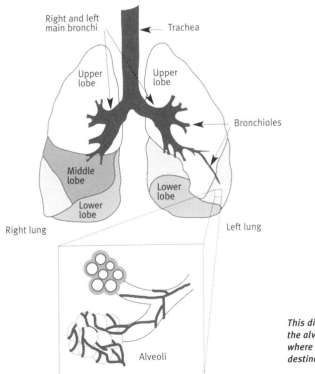

This diagram shows the alveloli, or air sacs where surfactant is destined to go.

Intracytoplasmic Sperm Injection (ICSI)

Severino Antinori (b. 1945)

The introduction of ICSI at the end of the 20th century provided hope to millions of infertile men, for whom previously the only solution had been to use donor sperm to achieve a pregnancy.

Using ICSI, a single sperm is injected into the egg, which has previously been collected and prepared using IVF. When the resulting fertilised egg develops into an early embryo it can then be reimplanted back into the woman.

The technique developed as a result of research by Severino Antorini, an Italian gynaecologist and embryologist. Antinori had originally been interested in gastroenterology, but retrained in obstetrics and gynaecology after he attended a lecture given by Patrick Steptoe (1913–1988) who was the first to successfully achieve a 'test-tube' baby using IVF in 1978.

Antinori set up his own clinic in Rome in 1982 and ten years later introduced ICSI as a technique to locate and implant a single, viable sperm directly into the egg. This technique has been successful even when there are virtually no sperm in the ejaculate.

Using a very small instrument to hold the egg steady, the embryologist uses a thin hollow needle to pierce the egg and inject a single sperm inside. The whole procedure is done under a microscope. Once the sperm is inside the egg, it's placed on a Petri dish filled with nutrients and checked the following day to see if it has been fertilized or not.

When ICSI was introduced there was some concern about an increased risk of birth defects associated with the technique. This is believed to be something to do with the selection of sperm that is different from the natural process.

In 2006, a modification to ICSI was introduced, allowing embryologists to choose more mature sperm for the procedure with the intention of lowering the risk of birth defects.

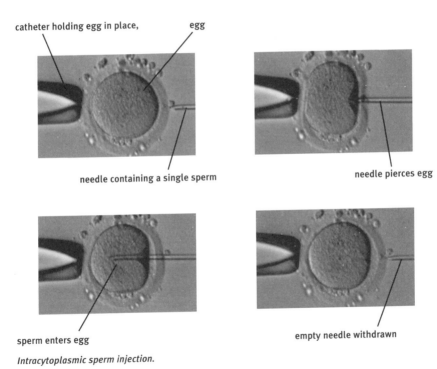

catheter holding egg in place,   egg

needle containing a single sperm

needle pierces egg

sperm enters egg

empty needle withdrawn

Intracytoplasmic sperm injection.

See: *In-Vitro Fertilization (IVF)*, pages 186–188

Combination Therapy for HIV Infection

The International Aids Society

When the media first described HIV infection, it was a rapidly fatal disease, a death sentence to anyone infected.

Since 1996, with the advent of combination therapy to treat HIV infection, many millions of people taking it have resumed a near normal life with a greatly extended life expectancy.

First reports of a new and unusual phenomenon in medicine came from America in 1981, when the *New York Times* reported an outbreak of a rare form of cancer among gay men in New York and California. At about the same time, there was also a sudden increase in the number of cases of young men presenting with a rare and severe pneumonia known as pneumocystis.

From these outbreaks spawned a worldwide epidemic of what we now know as HIV infection. The number of cases has spiralled, and the UNAIDS programme estimates that more than 40-million people are now infected, 70 per cent of them in sub-Saharan Africa.

The first patients to be diagnosed had a fairly quick demise. Estimates suggested that from diagnosis to death was a maximum of ten years. But progress in treatment has been equally rapid. By 1983, the HIV-virus had been identified and by the end of the decade a new treatment known as AZT emerged.

In the 1990s there was a rapid growth in the number of new drugs available to treat HIV but patients continued to be treated with one drug at a time, with limited success. At the end of 1995, the International AIDS Society convened an expert panel to come up with recommendations on how best to use these drugs. Its guidelines were first published in July 1996 to coincide with the Vancouver International AIDS Conference. The panel concluded that all the evidence pointed towards using combination therapy of three medicines together. These new 'triple therapies' might actually eliminate HIV infection, they claimed, and patients taking triple therapy would have an indefinite life expectancy with a good quality of life.

What seemed like a miracle – a cure for the HIV infection – almost happened. Unfortunately, the virus is still able to 'hide' in the body, making it impossible to completely get rid of it. But triple therapy has certainly increased life expectancy. And although these patients remain infectious, the treatment has provided renewed hope to millions of people who are now able to plan for a future they didn't think they had before.

Viagra®

*The introduction of Viagra marked a breakthrough
in the treatment of impotence.*

Before Viagra® was introduced there was no easy way of treating impotence. The only options were injections and vacuum pump devices which seemed an unattractive prospect to most men.

Viagra® was actually discovered by accident. The researchers at the pharmaceutical company Pfizer were concentrating on finding a new drug to treat angina. They were looking at drugs that target an enzyme in the arteries to keep them open more widely and, therefore, supply more oxygen to the heart. They found a drug, initially code-named UK–92,480, which looked promising and they progressed to research on healthy volunteer men.

The volunteers noticed that while the effect of UK–92, 480 on the coronary arteries was insufficient to make it useful in the treatment of angina, it did open up the arteries elsewhere in the body, particularly in the penis. An erection is achieved by blood flowing into the arteries, and UK–92, 480 made it possible for men who had previously had difficulty to establish and sustain an erection.

Impotence is a widespread but often not discussed subject. A recent survey among 1,000 UK-based men aged 18–75 showed that 39 per cent reported some form of erectile dysfunction while an estimated 30 million men in the United States suffer from the condition. Realizing they were onto something, the researchers at Pfizer switched their attention to using the drug to treat impotence.

The medicine, which came to be known as Sildenafil, and finally Viagra®, was tested in double-blind placebo-controlled trials starting in 1993. This meant neither researchers nor doctors knew which patients were receiving the drug and which were receiving only inactive placebo. Viagra® proved to be a great success and was given a licence so that doctors could prescribe it just six months after publication of the results of the research. 2.9 million prescriptions were written within three months!

Erectile dysfunction can be a symptom of many other serious conditions such as depression, diabetes, high blood pressure, heart disease and even prostate cancer. The publicity surrounding the introduction of Viagra® has meant that many new patients suffering with these conditions have consulted their doctor and received medical help.

Telesurgery

Jacques Marescaux (b. 1948)

*Using cutting-edge information technology,
a surgeon can now perform surgery on a patient
when they are in separate locations.*

During the procedure the surgeon holds dummy surgical instruments that control the position of the actual instruments in the patient. Meanwhile, the instruments operating on the patient are held by robots and respond to electronic messages received from the position of the surgeon's dummy instruments. All the time the surgeon receives visual images of the procedure showing the position of the instruments in the patient.

To be successful, this technique relies on reliable, high-speed transmission of images to and from the patient.

The first patient to receive telesurgery was a woman aged 68, who had her gall bladder removed using minimally invasive surgery. She was in an operating theatre in Strasbourg, with two surgeons standing by in case of a problem. Jacques Marescaux and his assistant surgeon were more than 7,000 km/4,350 mi away in New York. The 45-minute procedure was a success and many more procedures have been successfully completed since.

Telesurgery has potential for use in war zones because the technology allows surgeons to treat patients who may be on a contaminated or remote battlefield. It is also useful for treating patients who live a long way from good-quality medical care. In this situation, it may be possible for the patient to get to a telesurgery site where a doctor in another place could administer treatment.

Commenting on it, Marescaux said telesurgery lays the foundations *'for the globalization of surgical procedures, making it possible to imagine that a surgeon could perform an operation on a patient anywhere in the world'.*

Human Genome Project

The genome is the name given to the instructions in the DNA in each of our cells that make us the way we are.

Learning how to read the DNA code has been an enormous undertaking involving thousands of scientists all over the world for more than a decade.

Since James Watson and Francis Crick's discovery of the structure of DNA in 1953, scientists have been working towards understanding more about the genome.

The first step in the process was the discovery that the double helix of DNA is made up of two chains of alternating sugar and phosphate groups. Joining these two chains together into a twisted ladder shape, are 'rungs' made of four types of chemical, known as bases. The bases are adenine (A), cytosine (C), guanine (G), and thymine (T) and they can only be linked in certain combination. A can only link with T, C links with G, T with A, and G links with C.

The next step was to work out the sequence of the three billion base pairs in the 24 chromosomes found in every human cell.

Individual sections of DNA of differing lengths, otherwise known as genes, control part of a cells chemistry, particularly protein production. So once the sequence of base pairs had been identified, scientists turned to the task of identifying all the genes that code for a human: the genome.

Every person has their own individual sequence of genes, unless they have an identical twin. This has been useful for forensic science as a piece of DNA can help to identify a victim or confirm that a suspect has been at the scene of the crime.

Completing the Human Genome Project has been an enormous international collaboration. It marks the beginning of many new possibilities for understanding the genetic basis of disease, and for developing new treatments in the future.

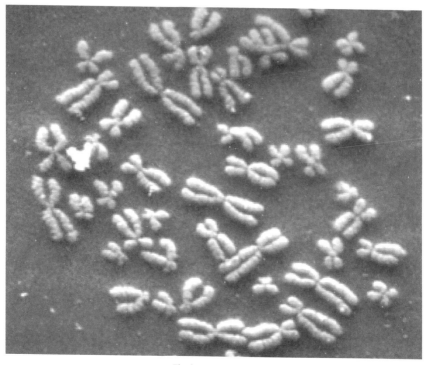

The human genome.

See: *The Structure of DNA*, pages 129–130

Eye Injections to Prevent Blindness

Philip J. Rosenfeld

When bevacizumab (Avastin®) was introduced in 2004 to treat advanced bowel cancer, some patients who had early eye disease noticed that their vision improved. It has since become a recognized treatment to prevent certain types of blindness.

Macular degeneration affects many older adults. The macula is important to central vision and when it doesn't function fully, it becomes harder to read or recognize faces.

The condition has two main types: dry and wet. In the dry form, the retina, which is the light sensitive lining at the back of the eye, deteriorates and becomes less able to detect images. In the wet form, many tiny new blood vessels grow into the area around the macular, damaging its ability to detect visual images. Diabetes can also cause damage to the blood vessels in the retina which then leak, resulting in a spongy waterlogged area around the macula.

Bevacizumab works by blocking the effect of a protein in the body called Vascular Endothelial Growth Factor (VEGF). In bowel cancer the treatment works by preventing the growth of new blood vessels that the tumour needs in order to grow and spread.

In the case of the eye, retinal damage also leads to the release of VEGF. New blood vessels form which lead to further damage to the area. Lasers are often used to treat this form of new blood vessel growth. But soon after the introduction of Avastin® onto the market, ophthalmologists realized that the same drug might stop new blood vessel growth in wet macular degeneration.

Philip Rosenfeld, professor of ophthalmology at the Bascom Palmer

Eye Institute, University of Miami Miller School of Medicine, Miami, Florida, was one of the first doctors to experiment with using Avastin® to treat macular degeneration with great success. Gradually more and more doctors began to do the same.

However, despite the emerging evidence that Avastin® is useful for preventing blindness, Genentech (the drug company that produces it) chose not to put this drug through the licensing process for use in ophthalmology, preferring instead to introduce two other more expensive drugs, Lucentis® and Macugen®. These both have a similar effect and are licensed for use in the eyes.

Although the injection sounds awful, it takes only a few seconds to do and usually feels like a tiny prick. The patient can go home the same day. It's often used in conjunction with laser therapy.

Eye Injection to treat wet macular degeneration.

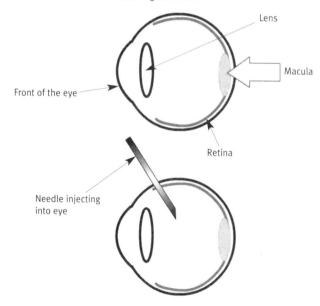

Lens

Macula

Front of the eye

Retina

Needle injecting into eye

Face Transplant

Bernard Devauchelle

Jean-Michel Dubernard

Medical breakthroughs are often accompanied by ethical debates, and none more so than in the case of face transplantation.

Although the technology to carry out a face transplant has been available since 1999, it took six years before the first operation took place.

The delay was as a result of ethical concerns, partly about the psychological impact on a patient of having the appearance of another person. However, doctors argued that the underlying bone structure of the recipient would be different from that of the donor, resulting in a 'hybrid' of both the donor and the recipient.

In the end the first transplant was carried out by a French team, led by Bernard Devauchelle and Jean-Michel Dubernard, ahead of rivals in the United States and United Kingdom.

The patient was 38-year old Isabelle Dinoire, from Valenciennes, north of Amiens in France, who had been mauled by her pet labrador and who had been unable to eat or speak properly since. She received a triangular flap of facial tissue containing the nose, lips and chin of a woman from Lille who had committed suicide hours earlier. Her family gave permission for the transplant after she was declared brain dead. The flap contained the muscles arteries and veins as well as the skin from the dead woman. Like any other transplant patient, Isabelle will have to take immunosuppressant drugs to avoid her body rejecting the donated face.

Doctors working in the field believe many more could benefit from the procedure, including 10,000 burns victims in the United Kingdom.

Computerized image of the transplant showing nerves, muscles and blood vessels.

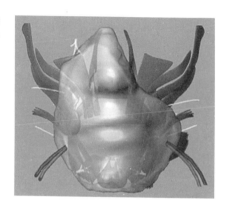

A model showing the area of the first face transplant.

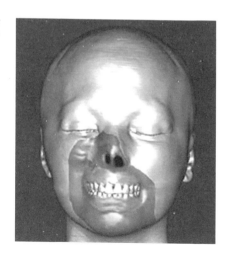

Cervical Cancer Vaccine

Ian Frazer (b. 1953)
Jian Zhou (1957–1999)

Gardasil® is the first vaccine designed to protect against certain types of wart virus infection, which are known to cause 70 per cent of cervical cancer cases.

Cervical cancer is the second most common cause of cancer deaths in women aged 15 to 44 across Europe, resulting in 275,000 deaths worldwide every year.

As little as 25 years ago, scientists didn't know what caused cervical cancer. Now it is well known that virtually all cases are caused by persistent infection with high-risk strains of the human papillomavirus or wart virus infection.

There are dozens of wart virus types, but only around 15 are high risk and can cause cervical cancer. There are also some types that cause genital warts. The vaccine protects against types 16 and 18, which cause 70 per cent of cervical cancer cases, and Types 6 and 11, which cause 90 per cent of genital warts cases.

A Scottish-born doctor, Ian Frazer, and a Chinese molecular virologist, Jian Zhou, invented the vaccine. They met in Cambridge and developed the vaccine at the University of Queensland in Australia.

The vaccine is designed to be given to young adults in their early teenage years, who are either not yet sexually active, or if they are, have not been infected with any or all of the virus types that cause warts and cancer. However, because it does not protect against all types of cervical cancer, it is still recommended that women have regular cervical smears.

Because it takes between 10–20 years for a cancer to develop after HPV infection, any benefits in relation to cervical cancer won't be seen for quite a long time.

Acknowledgements

As a teacher Roy Porter was flamboyant and inspirational. Before he died he gave us an immense contribution to the study of the History of Medicine, and I am fortunate to have been one of his students. His book, *The Greatest Benefit to Mankind, a Medical History of Humanity from Antiquity to the Present*, has been a valuable resource in the research for this book. I also acknowledge Mike Neve, Vivian Nutton, Bill Bynum, and Chris Lawrence, who along with Roy Porter taught me to understand the importance of historical context of modern day medicine. Their enormous combined wisdom has been a powerful influence in all of my writing. For teaching me to always reach for the highest standards in life, and for giving me confidence to remain open to new possibilities, I thank my parents Alma and Maurice and my sister Anna Craft.

References:

Page 22: *Traite de con uite de la famille, di Popozo*, Florentine Popozo,1829
Page 34: *A Treatise on the Scurvy*, Johann Bachstrom, 1753, Sands, Murray and Cochran for A Kincaid and A Donaldson
Page 36: 'A Dissertation on Artificial Teeth in General...', Nicholas Dubois De Chemant, 1797, J.Barker
Page 48: *The Autobiography of Charles Darwin*, Charles Darwin, John Murray, 1902
Page 89: *The Greatest Benefit to Mankind, a Medical History of Humanity from Antiquity to the Present*, Roy Porter, Fontana Press, 1997
Page 93: 'An Essay on the Recovery of the Apparently Dead', Charles Kite, London, 1788
Page 110: *Through the Iron Lung*, Mrs. V. A Pahl, Dryden Sinclair, 1955
Page 206: 'Surgeons perform operation across the Atlantic', Professor Marescaux, the *Telegraph*, 2001

Index

Index

Index